NTW NHS

NT06671

D1756241

Stroke Medicine

S.K. Gill • M.M. Brown • F. Robertson
N. Losseff
Editors

Stroke Medicine

Case Studies from Queen Square

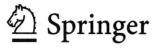 Springer

Editors
S.K. Gill
UCL Institute of Neurology Education Unit
National Hospital for Neurology
and Neurosurgery
London
UK

F. Robertson
Lysholm Department of Neuroradiology
National Hospital for Neurology
and Neurosurgery
London
UK

M.M. Brown
Brain Repair & Rehabilitation
UCL Institute of Neurology,
University College London
London
UK

N. Losseff
Department of Stroke
National Hospital for Neurology
and Neurosurgery
London
UK

ISBN 978-1-4471-6704-4   ISBN 978-1-4471-6705-1   (eBook)
DOI 10.1007/978-1-4471-6705-1

Library of Congress Control Number: 2015942706

Springer London Heidelberg New York Dordrecht

Printed on acid-free paper

Springer-Verlag London Ltd. is part of Springer Science+Business Media (www.springer.com)

For our patients.
-The Editors

Preface

The details of the case are important: their analysis distinguishes the expert from the journeyman. CM Fisher [1]

Learning through case analysis is a technique that centuries old and used in almost all disciplines. This 'storytelling' method of teaching adds layers of richness and a depth that can not be found in the linear structure of a standard textbook. The value of this – and the reason why we have chosen it for this book – is that it allows the reader the ability to view the thought processes involved in clinical decision-making. These 'grey cases' are often referred upward through the hierarchies of a specialty and can end up in tertiary centres where the diagnostic processes may be inexplicit. The aim of the book is to allow insight into the process of diagnosis and provide the tools to cut through the complexity inherent in neurovascular medicine to formulate a diagnosis and treatment plan. These are real cases, and it is important to recognise that despite the considerable experience of the physician it is possible that a alternative direction or treatment is followed before an answer is found. The discussion that follows each case describes the reasoning behind case management and highlights how an element of becoming a better physician means being open to exploring alternative possibilities. These cases also demonstrate how collaborative analysis of cases with other specialists increases the odds of good decision-making and that this is a vital skill to foster, in addition to being one of the most enjoyable aspects of clinical practice.

We hope that reading this book will add to your general clinical education as well as increase your depth of knowledge and understanding of neurovascular medicine. We have chosen cases that you are likely to come across as stroke physicians of the future and hope to leave you better equipped to problem-solve. In addition we hope this will inspire you to talk about your cases with your colleagues to explore clinical conundrums and enable you to resolve questions which often have no single right answer.

The structure of each chapter means that you are 'talked through' the case presentation and investigations. This is then followed by a thorough analysis with key learning points to highlight underlying principles. Imaging is included to illustrate the cases and we have also included radiological learning points. This book is a suitable companion for anyone from medical students through to experienced physicians to develop their knowledge and understanding of neurovascular medicine.

London, UK   Sumanjit K. Gill, BSc.hons, MBBS, MRCP
London, UK   Martin M. Brown, MA, MD, FRCP
London, UK   Fergus Robertson, MA, MD, MRCP, FRCR
London, UK   Nicholas Losseff, MD, FRCP

Reference

1. Caplan L. Fishers rules. Arch Neurol. 1982;39:389–90.

Contents

Contributors

Matthew Adams, MB BChir, FRCR Lysholm Department of Neuroradiology, National Hospital for Neurology and Neurosurgery, London, UK

Deepa Arachchillage, MRCP, FRCPath Haemostasis Research Unit, Department of Haematology, University College London Hospitals NHS Foundation Trust and University College London, London, UK

Asaipillai Asokanathan, MRCP (UK), DGM (London) Department of Stroke, East and North Hertfordshire NHS Trust, Stevenage, UK

Anish Bahra, FRCP, MD Department of Neurology, Bartshealth, Whipps Cross Hospital, London, UK and Department of Neurology, National Hospital for Neurology and Neurosurgery, London, UK

Pervinder Bhogal, MBBS, MRCS, FRCR, PG Dip MedEd Atkinson Morley Department of Neuroradiology, St. Georges Hospital, London, UK

Lucy Blair, MBChB, BMedSci Hyper Acute Stroke Unit, University College Hospital, London, London, UK

David Bradley, MRCPI, PhD Stroke and Acute Brain Injury Unit, National Hospital for Neurology and Neurosurgery, London, UK

Martin M. Brown, MA, MD, FRCP Stroke Research Group, Department of Brain Repair & Rehabilitation, UCL Institute of Neurology, University College London, The National Hospital for Neurology and Neurosurgery, London, UK

Nicholas F. Brown, MBBS, MA, MRCP Department of Neurology, Royal Free Hospital, London, London, UK

James R. Brown, FRCS Department of Vascular Surgery, Southend University Hospital, Southend on sea, Essex, UK

Andreas Charidimou, MD, MSc Stroke Research Group, Department of Brain Repair and Rehabilitation, UCL Institute of Neurology and National Hospital for Neurology and Neurosurgery, London, UK

Gerry Christofi, BSc, PhD, BM BCh, MRCP, MRCP Neurorehabilitation, National Hospital for Neurology and Neurosurgery, London, UK

Hannah Cohen, MD, FRCP, FRCPath Department of Haematology, University College London Hospitals NHS Foundation Trust and University College London, London, UK

David Collas, BSc, MBBS, FRCP Stroke Medicine, Watford General Hospital, Watford, UK

David Doig, MBChB, BScMedSci (Hons), MRCP Stroke Research Group, Department of Brain Repair and Rehabilitation, UCL Institute of Neurology, University College London and National Hospital for Neurology and Neurosurgery, London, UK

Daniel Epstein, MBCHB, MRCP Stroke Medicine, Barnet Hospital, Barnet Hertfordshire, UK

Rachel Farrell, MB BCh, MRCPI, PhD Neurorehabilitation, National Hospital for Neurology and Neurosurgery, UCLH, London, UK

Laura Flisher, BSs Hons, BSc Hons, HPC, CSP Therapies and Rehabilitation, National Hospital for Neurology and Neurosurgery, London, UK

Vijeya Ganesan, MRCPCH, MD Neurosciences Unit, UCL Institute of Child Health, London, UK

Sumanjit K. Gill, BSc Hons, MBBS, MRCP Education Unit, National Hospital for Neurology and Neurosurgery, UCL Institute of Neurology, London, UK

Lionel Ginsberg, BSc, MBBS, PhD, FRCP, FHEA Department of Neurology, Royal Free Hospital, London, UK

Joan P. Grieve, MD, FRCS (SN) Department of Neurosurgery, National Hospital for Neurology and Neurosurgery, London, UK

Paul Guyler, MRCP Acute Stroke Medicine, Southend University Hospital, Southend on sea, Essex, UK

Jeremy C.S. Johnson, MBBS, BSc Department of Stroke, National Hospital for Neurology and Neurosurgery, London, UK

Fiona Kennedy, MB, Bch, BAO, MRCP (UK) Stroke Research Group, Department of Brain Repair and Rehabilitation, UCL Institute of Neurology, University College London and National Hospital for Neurology and Neurosurgery, London, UK

Ashvini Keshavan, MB, BChir Department of Brain Repair and Rehabilitation, UCL Institute of Neurology, University College London and National Hospital for Neurology and Neurosurgery, London, UK

Ruth Law, MA, MBBS, MRCP Department of Medicine, University College London, London, UK

Alexander Leff, PhD, FRCP Institute of Cognitive Neuroscience and Department of Brain Repair and Rehabilitation, UCL Institute of Neurology, University College London and National Hospital for Neurology and Neurosurgery, London, UK

Thaya Loganathan, MRCP Acute Stroke Medicine, Southend University Hospital, Southend on sea, Essex, UK

Nicholas Losseff, MD, FRCP Department of Stroke, The National Hospital for Neurology and Neurosurgery, London, UK

Robert I. Luder, BSc (Hons), FRCP (UK) Department of Stroke Medicine, North Middlesex University Hospital, Edmonton, London, UK

Ari Manuel, MBBS, MRCP, BSc, DipLATHE Oxford Sleep Unit, Oxford University Hospitals NHS Trust, Oxford, Oxfordshire, UK

Áine Merwick, MB, BMed Sc, MSc, PhD, MRCPI Department of Neurology, National Hospital for Neurology and Neurosurgery, Queen Square, London, UK

Kelvin Kuan Huei Ng, MBBS Stroke Neurology Department, Hamilton General Hospital, Hamilton, ON, Canada

Georgios Niotakis Paediatric Neurology, Great Ormond Street Hospital for Children, London, UK

Anthony O'Brien, MRCP Acute Stroke Medicine, Southend University Hospital, Southend on sea, Essex, UK

Rupert Oliver, PhD, MRCP Department of Neurology, Guy's and St. Thomas' Hospitals, St. Thomas' Hospital, London, UK

Richard Perry, BM, BCh, MA, PhD, MRCP (UK) Department of Neurology, National Hospital for Neurology & Neurosurgery, London, UK

Menelaos Pipis, MBBS, BSc (Hons), MRCP Department of Medicine, Northwick Park Hospital, Harrow, Middlesex, London, UK

Stefanie Christina Robert, MD, MRCP, FFICM Intensive Care Unit, Homerton University Hospital, London, UK

Anne Jutta Schmitt, Dr. Med. Univ. Department of Radiology, University College London Hospital, London, UK

Raja Farhat Shoaib, MRCPS Acute Stroke Medicine, Southend University Hospital, Southend on sea, Essex, UK

Robert Simister, MA, FRCP, PhD Comprehensive Stroke Service, National Hospital for Neurology and Neurosurgery, UCLH Trust, London, UK

Devesh Sinha, MRCP Acute Stroke Medicine, Southend University Hospital, Southend on sea, Essex, UK

Shaun Ude, MRCP Acute Stroke Medicine, Southend University Hospital, Southend on sea, Essex, UK

David J. Werring, BSc, MBBS, PhD, FRCP Stroke Research Group, Department of Brain Repair and Rehabilitation, UCL Institute of Neurology and National Hospital for Neurology and Neurosurgery, London, UK

Victoria Wykes, MB, PhD, MRCS Department of Neurosurgery, National Hospital for Neurology and Neurosurgery, London, UK

Chapter 1
A Rapidly Progressive Dementia

Andreas Charidimou and David J. Werring

Clinical History

A 76-year old man presented following a brief episode of collapse whilst on the train. He remembered feeling unwell, and then waking up on the train surrounded by people, having briefly lost consciousness. He reported no chest pain, nor any markers of seizure activity. Prior to this event he had suffered progressive cognitive decline over at least 6 months, with difficulties with memory, concentration and sustained attention. During his inpatient stay, the patient became more confused with worsening cognitive impairment, frequent disorientation in time and place, inappropriate behaviour and wandering.

He had a past medical history of hypertension, a right frontal intracerebral haemorrhage (ICH) associated with a fall 2 years before current presentation, and a previous ischaemic stroke causing left hemianopia.

Examination

The cranial nerves were normal apart from longstanding left homonymous hemianopia. Reflexes were symmetrical with flexor plantar responses and there was no limb weakness or sensory deficits. Neuropsychological assessment demonstrated impaired recognition memory, executive function, cognitive speed, attention, and nominal skills.

A. Charidimou, MD, MSc (✉) • D.J. Werring, BSc, MBBS, PhD, FRCP (✉)
Stroke Research Group, Department of Brain Repair and Rehabilitation, UCL Institute
of Neurology and National Hospital for Neurology and Neurosurgery, London, UK
e-mail: a.charidimou@ucl.ac.uk; d.werring@ucl.ac.uk

© Springer-Verlag London 2015
S.K. Gill et al. (eds.), *Stroke Medicine: Case Studies from Queen Square*,
DOI 10.1007/978-1-4471-6705-1_1

1

Investigations

A non-contrast CT of the brain demonstrated an established right temporal-occipital infarct and volume loss in the right frontal lobe. CT angiography showed no evidence of an arteriovenous malformation or other vascular abnormality. A brain MRI scan including T2*-weighted gradient-recalled echo (T2*-GRE) and susceptibility-weighted imaging (SWI) showed multiple strictly lobar cerebral microbleeds, predominantly in the occipital and temporal lobes, extensive superficial cortical haemosiderin staining, and a previous ICH in the right frontal lobe. There were also severe confluent and patchy white matter hyperintensities (leukoaraiosis) and an area of encephalomalacia consistent with a mature infarct in the right temporal-occipital lobe. Representative images are shown in Fig. 1.1.

Routine blood tests including biochemistry, renal, liver, and bone profiles, full blood count, and CRP were normal; the autoimmune screen was negative. Lumbar puncture was performed, and analysis revealed clear cerebrospinal fluid (CSF). Glucose was normal; the protein level was mildly elevated (0.73 g/L; normal range: 0.13–0.40 g/L) without pleocytosis (<1 white cell, <1 red cell; only occasional small mature lymphocytes and rare macrophages). CSF 14-3-3 protein was negative. Electroencephalogram (EEG) recording on two occasions showed generalized slowing of background rhythms but no epileptiform activity.

The patient remained extremely confused, with inappropriate behaviour, while his cognitive function continued to decline. A diagnosis of severe cerebral amyloid angiopathy (CAA) was suspected and the patient had a non-dominant (right) frontal brain biopsy to confirm the diagnosis and exclude any treatable pathology. Neuropathology confirmed severe CAA in the leptomeninges and cerebral cortex. Routine haematoxylin and eosin (H&E) stain showed circumferential thickening and

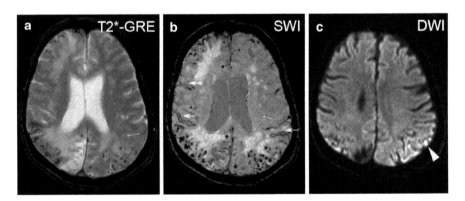

Fig. 1.1 (**a**) T2*-weighted gradient-recalled echo (*T2*-GRE*) MRI shows numerous lobar cerebral microbleeds particularly in posterior brain regions characteristic of cerebral amyloid angiopathy. (**b**) Susceptibility-weighted imaging (*SWI*) shows even more numerous cerebral microbleeds and extensive cortical superficial siderosis involving multiple cerebral sulci (*black serpiginous lines*; *arrowed*). Marked confluent and patchy white matter hyperintensities (leukoaraiosis) are also evident. (**c**) Diffusion weighted imaging (*DWI*) shows a small hyperintense lesion (*arrowhead*) consistent with an acute ischaemic lesion in the left parietal lobe ("microinfarct")

amorphous eosinophilic appearance of leptomeningeal, cortical and to lesser extent white matter blood vessels with conspicuous loss of smooth muscle cells. This was accompanied, particularly in the leptomeninges, by patchy cracking and "double-barrelling" of the vessel walls. Immunohistochemistry confirmed widespread amyloid-β deposition within the leptomeningeal and cortical blood vessels, including capillaries. There was no evidence of either prion protein or vasculitis (Fig. 1.2).

The patient was treated with antihypertensives and donepezil (a centrally acting reversible acetylcholinesterase inhibitor), but his cognition and behaviour continued to progressively deteriorate.

Discussion

Sporadic CAA is a common age-related cerebral small vessel disease, characterised by progressive deposition of amyloid-β in the wall of small cortical and leptomeningeal arteries [1]. Population-based autopsy studies show that the prevalence of CAA is 20–40% in non-demented, and 50–60% in demented elderly populations [2, 3]. Deposition of amyloid-β causes injury to the vessel wall, which in moderate to severe disease may rupture, causing cerebral microbleeds, cortical superficial siderosis or larger symptomatic ICH [4]. Amyloid-β deposits can also narrow or occlude vessel lumen, potentially causing cerebral ischaemia (cerebral infarction, "microinfarcts" or leukoaraiosis) [5]. The cause of CAA is not known. Conventional vascular risk factors do not seem to play a major causal role. Although some genetic risk factors (especially the apolipoprotein E e4 allele) are robustly associated with CAA, age remains the most powerful risk factor [4].

Although CAA is most often recognized by the occurrence of spontaneous lobar ICH in the elderly, it can also cause transient focal neurological deficits, disturbances of consciousness, and progressive cognitive decline [4, 6].

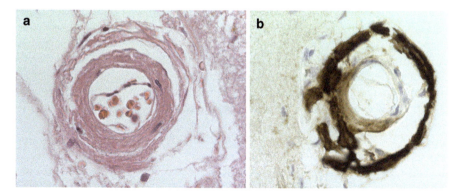

Fig. 1.2 (**a**) Haematoxylin and eosin (H&E) stain showing thickening and amorphous eosinophilic appearance of leptomeningeal small blood vessels with double barrelling of the vessel walls. (**b**) Immunohistochemistry showing severe amyloid-β deposition within a leptomeningeal vessel (*brown*), with double barrelling and patchy cracking

Symptomatic, spontaneous, lobar intracerebral haemorrhage in elderly patients is the most common clinical manifestation of CAA [4, 6]. The majority of intracerebral haemorrhages (>75%) in the elderly are spontaneous (non-traumatic), attributed to resulting from rupture of small arteries affected by two main processes: hypertensive arteriopathy (characterised by lipohyalinosis and fibrinoid necrosis of small lenticulostriate arterial perforators) or CAA (characterised by vascular amyloid-β deposits in the cortex and subcortical white matter). CAA accounts for up to 20% of spontaneous ICH in elderly subjects; CAA-related ICH are typically lobar, due to the distribution of the arterial pathology, and characterized by frequently early recurrence or synchronous multiple haemorrhages. By contrast, deep or infratentorial ICH (e.g. basal ganglia, thalamus and pons) are characteristic of hypertensive arteriopathy haemorrhage. There is also an association between CAA and anticoagulation or thrombolysis related ICH [7–9].

CAA is also associated with transient focal neurological episodes (sometime called "amyloid spells"), which can resemble transient ischaemic attacks, migraine auras or focal seizures [10–12]. Patients often complain of recurrent, brief (minutes), stereotyped attacks of paresthesias or numbness (spreading smoothly over contiguous body parts), visual symptoms (sometimes migraine aura-like), face or limb weakness or dysphasia. Although these symptoms may clinically suggest transient ischaemic attacks, increasing data suggest that "amyloid spells" in CAA are more often associated with intracranial bleeding (especially cortical superficial siderosis or focal convexity subarachnoid haemorrhage on T2*-GRE MRI) and a high early risk of symptomatic lobar ICH (24.5% [95% CI: 15.8–36.9%] at 8 weeks) [10]. Thus, antithrombotic drugs should generally be avoided in these patients due to the risk of serious future ICH [13].

There is increasing evidence that CAA is an important cause of cognitive impairment and dementia, although dissecting its independent impact is confounded by coexisting Alzheimer's disease and other age-related cerebrovascular pathologies [3]. Nearly all cases of Alzheimer's disease show CAA, while patients with CAA usually have some evidence of parenchymal amyloid. However, by contrast with Alzheimer's disease, the dementia associated with CAA typically progresses rapidly, usually with both large and small areas of haemorrhage and infarction, and prominent white matter abnormality (leukoaraiosis). Although it is difficult to attribute the rapid cognitive decline to any particular pathological component, the Religious Orders Study autopsy series found that moderate-to-severe CAA was associated with lower performance in specific cognitive domains after adjusting for Alzheimer's disease pathology and other potential confounders, notably perceptual speed and episodic memory [14].

A distinctly rare but clinically aggressive form of CAA is that of CAA-related inflammation (also termed cerebral amyloid angiitis, amyloid-β related angiitis and cerebral amyloid inflammatory vasculopathy) [15], characterized histopathologically by vascular or perivascular inflammatory infiltrates associated with amyloid-β laden vessels [16, 17]. CAA-related inflammation typically presents with acute cognitive decline, behavioural changes, seizures, headache, and focal neurologic deficits [15]. Neuroimaging typically reveals a potentially reversible leukoencephalopathy consisting of patchy or confluent, usually asymmetric white matter changes, sometimes with mass effect and contrast-enhancement, lobar ICH and multiple strictly lobar cerebral microbleeds on T2*-GRE MRI sequences (Fig. 1.1) [15]. The syndrome may respond to corticosteroids or other immuno-modulatory treatment. CAA-related inflammation is similar to that observed in patients with Alzheimer's disease who developed meningo-encephalitis after immunisation against human amyloid-β (ARIA: Amyloid-Related Imaging Abnormalities) [16–19], which may relate to rapid movement of amyloid from brain parenchyma into blood vessels [20, 21].

The "gold standard" for definitive diagnosis of CAA remains histopathological analysis, usually from haematoma evacuation or brain biopsy and, less commonly, brain autopsy [22]. However, the radiological demonstration of haemorrhagic mani-festations of the disease in the brain (especially using T2*-GRE or SWI MRI) allow the *in vivo* clinical-radiological diagnosis of CAA. The diagnosis of CAA currently relies on the demonstration of multiple haemorrhagic lesions in strictly lobar brain areas – the "Boston criteria", including both cerebral micro-bleeds, as well as ICH, although pathological validation for microbleed-only patients is limited [22–24]. Cerebral microbleeds are small, dark, rounded areas detected on blood-sensitive MRI sequences that seem to reflect small areas of bleeding from fragile vessels affected by small vessel disease including CAA [25]. The detection of cortical superficial siderosis as in our patient, possibly reflecting repeated episodes of bleed-ing into the subarachnoid space and over the surface of the brain seems to another characteristic imaging feature of CAA [23].

In summary, our case represents a progressive dementia due to severe CAA, a common but under-recognized form of cerebral small vessel disease. Our case illus-trates the characteristic clinical and neuroimaging spectrum of CAA and the impor-tant role of advanced brain MRI including blood-sensitive sequence for investigation and *in vivo* diagnosis. As populations age, CAA is likely to become an increasingly important cause of disability in stroke medicine. With the prospect of disease-modifying treatments to reduce vascular amyloid deposition [4], as well as effective treatment of all known risk factors (including hypertension), making the correct diagnosis of CAA will become increasingly important.

Key Clinical Learning Points
1. CAA is a common age-related cerebral small vessel disease
2. It is caused by amyloid-β deposition in small cortical and leptomeningeal arteries
3. CAA is commonly associated with lobar intracerebral haemorrhage in elderly patients
4. CAA can also present with transient focal neurological symptoms or progressive cognitive impairment and dementia
5. CAA-related inflammation is an uncommon but distinctly aggressive sub-type of CAA, which typically presents with acute cognitive decline, behavioural change, seizures, headache, and focal neurologic deficits

Key Radiological Learning Points
1. CAA diagnosis relies on neuroimaging demonstration of multiple areas of strictly lobar cerebral haemorrhage (Boston criteria)
2. Characteristic imaging correlates on blood-sensitive MRI sequences (including T2*-GRE or SWI) include strictly lobar cerebral microbleeds, ICH and cortical superficial siderosis
3. Other imaging findings in CAA include white matter hyperintensities (leukoaraiosis) and small or large areas of cerebral infarction, including apparently clinically silent "microinfarcts"

References

1. Vinters HV. Cerebral amyloid angiopathy. A critical review. Stroke. 1987;18(2):311–24. Epub 1987/03/01.
2. Keage HA, Carare RO, Friedland RP, et al. Population studies of sporadic cerebral amyloid angiopathy and dementia: a systematic review. BMC Neurol. 2009;9:3. Epub 2009/01/16.
3. MRC CFAS. Pathological correlates of late-onset dementia in a multicentre, community-based population in England and Wales. Neuropathology Group of the Medical Research Council Cognitive Function and Ageing Study (MRC CFAS). Lancet. 2001;357(9251):169–75. Epub 2001/02/24.
4. Charidimou A, Gang Q, Werring DJ. Sporadic cerebral amyloid angiopathy revisited: recent insights into pathophysiology and clinical spectrum. J Neurol Neurosurg Psychiatry. 2012;83(2):124–37. Epub 2011/11/08.
5. Smith EE, Schneider JA, Wardlaw JM, et al. Cerebral microinfarcts: the invisible lesions. Lancet Neurol. 2012;11(3):272–82. Epub 2012/02/22.
6. Viswanathan A, Greenberg SM. Cerebral amyloid angiopathy in the elderly. Ann Neurol. 2011;70(6):871–80. Epub 2011/12/23.
7. Rosand J, Hylek EM, O'Donnell HC, et al. Warfarin-associated hemorrhage and cerebral amyloid angiopathy: a genetic and pathologic study. Neurology. 2000;55(7):947–51. Epub 2000/11/04.
8. Sloan MA, Price TR, Petito CK, et al. Clinical features and pathogenesis of intracerebral hemorrhage after rt-PA and heparin therapy for acute myocardial infarction: the Thrombolysis in Myocardial Infarction (TIMI) II Pilot and Randomized Clinical Trial combined experience. Neurology. 1995;45(4):649–58. Epub 1995/04/01.
9. McCarron MO, Nicoll JA. Cerebral amyloid angiopathy and thrombolysis-related intracerebral haemorrhage. Lancet Neurol. 2004;3(8):484–92. Epub 2004/07/21.
10. Charidimou A, Peeters A, Fox Z, et al. Spectrum of transient focal neurological episodes in cerebral amyloid angiopathy: multicentre magnetic resonance imaging cohort study and meta-analysis. Stroke. 2012;43(9):2324–30. Epub 2012/07/17.
11. Greenberg SM, Vonsattel JPG, Stakes JW, et al. The clinical spectrum of cerebral amyloid angiopathy: presentations without lobar hemorrhage. Neurology. 1993;43(10):2073–9.
12. Charidimou A, Law R, Werring DJ. Amyloid "spells" trouble. Lancet. 2012;380(9853):1620. Epub 2012/11/06.
13. Charidimou A, Baron JC, Werring DJ. Transient focal neurological episodes, cerebral amyloid angiopathy, and intracerebral hemorrhage risk: looking beyond TIAs. Int J Stroke. 2013;8(2):105–8. Epub 2013/01/23.

14. Arvanitakis Z, Leurgans SE, Wang Z, et al. Cerebral amyloid angiopathy pathology and cognitive domains in older persons. Ann Neurol. 2011;69(2):320–7. Epub 2011/03/10.
15. Chung KK, Anderson NE, Hutchinson D, et al. Cerebral amyloid angiopathy related inflammation: three case reports and a review. J Neurol Neurosurg Psychiatry. 2011;82(1): 20–6. Epub 2010/10/12.
16. Eng JA, Frosch MP, Choi K, et al. Clinical manifestations of cerebral amyloid angiopathy-related inflammation. Ann Neurol. 2004;55(2):250–6. Epub 2004/02/03.
17. Scolding NJ, Joseph F, Kirby PA, et al. Abeta-related angiitis: primary angiitis of the central nervous system associated with cerebral amyloid angiopathy. Brain. 2005;128(Pt 3):500–15. Epub 2005/01/22.
18. Sperling R, Salloway S, Brooks DJ, et al. Amyloid-related imaging abnormalities in patients with Alzheimer's disease treated with bapineuzumab: a retrospective analysis. Lancet Neurol. 2012;11(3):241–9. Epub 2012/02/07.
19. Sperling RA, Jack Jr CR, Black SE, et al. Amyloid-related imaging abnormalities in amyloid-modifying therapeutic trials: recommendations from the Alzheimer's Association Research Roundtable Workgroup. Alzheimers Dement. 2011;7(4):367–85. Epub 2011/07/26.
20. Nicoll JA, Wilkinson D, Holmes C, et al. Neuropathology of human Alzheimer disease after immunization with amyloid-beta peptide: a case report. Nat Med. 2003;9(4):448–52. Epub 2003/03/18.
21. Ferrer I, Boada Rovira M, Sanchez Guerra ML, et al. Neuropathology and pathogenesis of encephalitis following amyloid-beta immunization in Alzheimer's disease. Brain Pathol. 2004;14(1):11–20. Epub 2004/03/05.
22. Knudsen KA, Rosand J, Karluk D, Greenberg SM. Clinical diagnosis of cerebral amyloid angiopathy: validation of the Boston criteria. Neurology. 2001;56(4):537–9. Epub 2001/02/27.
23. Linn J, Halpin A, Demaerel P, et al. Prevalence of superficial siderosis in patients with cerebral amyloid angiopathy. Neurology. 2010;74(17):1346–50. Epub 2010/04/28.
24. van Rooden S, van der Grond J, van den Boom R, et al. Descriptive analysis of the Boston criteria applied to a Dutch-type cerebral amyloid angiopathy population. Stroke. 2009;40(9):3022–7. Epub 2009/06/27.
25. Greenberg SM, Vernooij MW, Cordonnier C, et al. Cerebral microbleeds: a guide to detection and interpretation. Lancet Neurol. 2009;8(2):165–74. Epub 2009/01/24.

Chapter 2
A Headache After Starting the Oral Contraceptive Pill

Matthew Adams

Clinical History

An 18-year-old right-handed female student collapsed at home and was transferred to the Accident and Emergency Department of the local hospital by ambulance. She described a 5-day history of severe, progressively worsening generalised headache and reported that just prior to her collapse she developed left lower limb weakness. She then noticed that she had blurred vision, worse on lateral gaze, and a left sided hemisensory disturbance. She gave a past medical history of two spontaneous miscarriages and had recently started taking the oral contraceptive pill.

Examination

She was alert and orientated. Her temperature was 37.2 °C, blood pressure 154/70 mmHg and her pulse was regular. There were no rashes or clinical evidence of meningism. Her pupils were equal and reactive, there was no conjunctival injection, visual fields were normal to confrontation and eye movements were normal. Fundoscopy revealed bilateral early papilloedema, worse on the right. She had a mild left pronator drift, mild weakness of shoulder abduction and hip flexion (MRC score 4) and an extensor plantar response on the left. Sensory assessment was normal, as was a general physical examination.

M. Adams, MB BChir, FRCR
Lysholm Department of Neuroradiology,
National Hospital for Neurology and Neurosurgery, London, UK
e-mail: matthew.adams@uclh.nhs.uk

© Springer-Verlag London 2015
S.K. Gill et al. (eds.), *Stroke Medicine: Case Studies from Queen Square*,
DOI 10.1007/978-1-4471-6705-1_2

Investigations

Blood samples sent on arrival in casualty showed normal full blood count, renal and liver profiles. D-Dimer was significantly elevated.

A plain CT brain demonstrated abnormal high attenuation within the straight sinus, vein of Galen and right internal cerebral vein, all of which were markedly expanded (Fig. 2.1). Low attenuation was seen throughout the lentiform nucleus, caudate head, capsular white matter and anterior thalamus on the right with moderate associated swelling. There was no evidence of subarachnoid blood and the ventricles were not enlarged. MRI revealed abnormal signal, swelling and petechial haemorrhage within the deep grey nuclei, capsular and periventricular frontal white matter and splenium of the corpus callosum on the right (Fig. 2.2). Occlusive thrombus within the straight sinus, vein of Galen and right internal cerebral vein was seen as abnormally high signal and expansion of the vessels on the T1-weighted imaging (Fig. 2.3), absence of the normal flow voids on the T2-weighted sequences and abnormally low signal and exaggeration of vessel calibre on susceptibility weighted imaging (SWI-blood sensitive sequence with features in common with T2*-weighted imaging). MR venography confirmed absent flow.

Ophthalmological assessment showed papilloedema but normal visual acuity and fields.

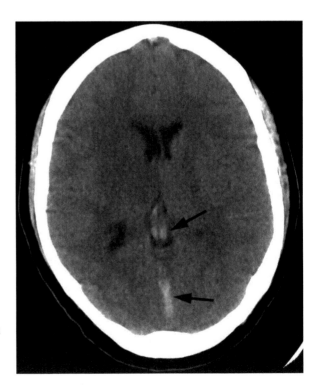

Fig. 2.1 CT showing high attenuation thrombus within distended internal cerebral veins and straight sinus (*arrows*) and low attenuation within the right lentiform nucleus, caudate head and thalamus on the right

A diagnosis was made of cerebral venous thrombosis involving the deep cerebral veins. Anticoagulation with low molecular weight heparin was commenced. She was discharged from hospital on oral anticoagulation and

Fig. 2.2 T2-weighted axial image demonstrating swelling and abnormal signal throughout the lentiform nucleus, caudate head, thalamus, capsular white matter and genu of the corpus callosum on the right extending to the frontal periventricular white matter

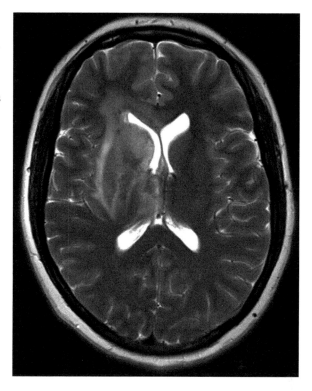

Fig. 2.3 T1-weighted sagittal image showing hyperintense thrombus within the straight sinus and internal cerebral vein (*arrow*)

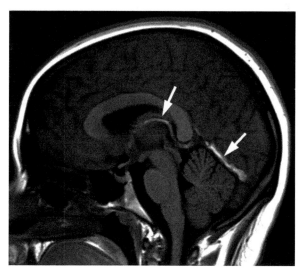

acetazolamide. Arrangements were made for serial assessment of visual function. A subsequent thrombophilia screen revealed the presence of antiphospholipid antibodies. Follow up imaging at 6 months showed resolution of the thrombosis.

Discussion

Cerebral venous sinus thrombosis (CVT) is an uncommon disorder with an annual incidence of 2–7 cases per million [1] and accounts for 0.5–1% of strokes. It more commonly affects younger patients, with over 75% occurring in those under 50 years of age [2]. With prompt diagnosis and appropriate therapy, the majority of patients make a good recovery, with poor neurological outcome seen in 7–20% of cases [3].

CVT typically presents with findings related to raised intracranial pressure and/ or the more focal effects of venous ischaemia or haemorrhage. Headache is the most common presenting symptom, typically diffuse and progressively worsening but occasionally thunderclap. CVT is an important cause of isolated intracranial hypertension ("benign" intracranial hypertension). However, in the context of patients presenting with stroke, the region of brain affected by venous ischaemia or haemorrhage determines the more focal clinical manifestations and is influenced by location of the thrombosis, which frequently involves multiple sites. With cortical involvement, as may occur in superior sagittal, transverse sinus or cortical vein thrombosis, there may be seizures, motor deficits, or aphasia. The classical clinical triad of headache, seizures and focal motor deficit should prompt early consideration of the diagnosis. Bilateral signs and gradually deteriorating symptoms are also relatively common features and may help to discriminate venous from arterial ischaemia. With thrombosis of the deep venous system (internal cerebral veins, basal vein of Rosenthal and vein of Galen), the archetypal presentation is depressed consciousness and diencephalic dysfunction; however, partial syndromes with preserved consciousness and focal symptoms, including hemiparesis and visual field defects are well recognised [4].

Although 15–20% of cases are unprovoked, numerous acquired and genetic factors have been shown to predispose to CVT. Prothrombotic states, especially thrombophilia caused by inherited deficiencies of proteins C and S or mutations of the genes encoding factor V Leiden and prothrombin G20210A are all well recognised risk factors. There is also an association with antiphospholipid antibodies. There is often a precipitating factor e.g. dehydration acting with another predisposing factor. The incidence of CVT increases during pregnancy due to a transient prothrombotic state that persists for 1–2 months post partum and may be exacerbated at the time of delivery by dehydration. Oral contraceptives are also a predisposing factor as in this case, with the risk being greater in those women with hereditary prothrombotic conditions. The presence of cancer, particularly myeloproliferative neoplasia, is also associated with increased risk. Less common causes include sinus trauma, parameningeal infections (especially otitis media and mastoiditis), particularly in the paediatric population, and systemic diseases, including inflammatory bowel disease and Behcets disease [2].

The investigation of suspected CVT should include full blood count and assessment of prothrombin time and activated partial thromboplastin time. D-Dimer levels are usually abnormally high in CVT but false negatives are well recognised, particularly in subacute or chronic presentations, and a normal assay should not discourage further investigation if clinical suspicion is high. Screening for genetic and acquired thrombophilia is required, but abnormal levels of antithrombin III, protein C and S should be tested after cessation of anticoagulation. Positive antiphospholipid antibodies require confirmatory repeat assays and specialist haematology assessment as false positives due to transiently high titres are relatively common. Investigation for mutation of the JAK2 gene, a specific marker of myeloproliferative neoplasia, should also be considered. Examination and follow up by an ophthalmologist is required for patients with papilloedema or visual symptoms [2]. If vision deteriorates despite medical treatment of CVT, optic nerve decompression may be required.

Both CT and MRI are useful non-invasive imaging modalities but routine structural imaging has a limited sensitivity in isolation and should be combined with CT or MR venography when clinical suspicion of CVT is high. The parenchymal changes of venous ischaemia appear as low attenuation regions and are frequently haemorrhagic. They may be bilateral, particularly if the superior sagittal sinus or deep venous system is involved. The finding of ischaemia or infarction that does not respect a typical arterial territory is very suggestive of the diagnosis (Fig. 2.2). Patchy haemorrhage within an infarct that suggests haemorrhagic transformation, but is seen on the first CT or MRI done within the first few hours after onset, is also indicative of venous thrombosis. Another clue may be that the patient does not have as extensive a focal deficit as one would expect from the apparent extent of the abnormality on parenchymal imaging. The secondary parenchymal changes of venous infarction are better demonstrated by MRI than CT. T2*-weighted and SWI sequences are very sensitive in detecting associated parenchymal and subarachnoid haemorrhage. The parenchymal appearances on diffusion-weighted imaging are variable and can reflect either vasogenic oedema, cytotoxic oedema or a combination of the two. Lesions with increased diffusion are more likely to resolve without parenchymal sequelae although even areas of restricted diffusion may be reversible [5].

The principle role of subsequent imaging is to demonstrate the venous thrombosis itself and the secondary effects on the brain parenchyma. Non-contrast CT is positive in approximately one third of cases [2]. In the early stages, thrombosed dural sinuses or veins appear hyperdense but the intensity on CT reduces as the clot matures and attenuation values decrease. CT venography improves sensitivity by highlighting clot as luminal filling defects or showing isolated enhancement of the dural wall when the sinus is completely occluded. Clot within the superior sagittal sinus, the most common site of CVT, gives rise to the so-called 'delta sign' due its triangular profile in CT axial section and the inverse 'empty delta sign' on venography due to enhancement of its dural margins.

Detection of venous thrombus on MRI is complicated by the fact that signal characteristics of clot fluctuate over time and because normal venous structures also have a variable signal due to the effects of flowing blood. The signal intensity of venous thrombus varies according to the interval between formation and imaging, principally reflecting the decomposition of haemoglobin. In the acute stage (0–5 days), deoxyhaemoglobin results in isointense and hypointense signal on T1 and T2-weighted imaging respectively and may mimic normal flow states, making detection of the clot particularly challenging. In the subacute stage (6–15 days), methaemoglobin results in high signal on both T1 and T2-weighted images and is the most straightforward to detect. The signal from chronic thrombus is variable but usually isointense on T1-weighted and isointense or hyperintense on T2-weighted images [1]. Chronic thrombus may also enhance and be difficult to distinguish from the luminal enhancement of a normal patent sinus. Sequences such as T2*-weighted ('gradient echo') and susceptibility weighted imaging (SWI) are very sensitive to the presence of paramagnetic blood components and can be used as an adjunct to the standard T1 and T2-weighted sequences. Intense signal loss with a 'blooming' effect often results in thrombosed vessels appearing more expanded than on other sequences and may be particularly useful in identifying cortical or deep vein thrombosis [6]. As with CTV, contrast enhanced MRI can be used to highlight luminal filling defects. MR venography can be used to show lack of flow in the occluded vessels and is particularly important in discriminating acute thrombus from normal flow states.

The mainstay of CVT treatment is unfractionated or low molecular weight heparin followed by oral vitamin K antagonists. This has been shown to be safe and probably effective in the adult population [2, 3, 7] and is not contraindicated by intraparenchymal haemorrhage at presentation [2, 3]. Due to the lack of adequate trial data, the optimum duration of oral anticoagulation is not known. However, where a transient risk factor is identified it is reasonable to limit treatment to 3–6 months, but if the CVT is unprovoked or there is mild thrombophilia treatment is usually continued for 6–12 months, guided by repeat venography. Indefinite anticoagulation should be considered in severe thrombophilia, malignancy or recurrent thrombosis [2, 3]. Long-term anticoagulation should also be considered if follow up imaging shows persistent stenosis of the affected venous sinus. Endovascular clot disruption or thrombolysis may have role if a patient deteriorates on anticoagulation but evidence is limited. Acetazolamide is a reasonable adjunct in patients presenting with intracranial hypertension and interventions such as therapeutic lumbar puncture, CSF shunting and optic nerve sheath fenestration may be considered in those with progressive visual failure [2].

Key Clinical Learning Points
1. CVT typically presents with findings related to raised intracranial pressure and/or the more focal effects of venous ischaemia or haemorrhage
2. Bilateral signs, seizures and gradually deteriorating symptoms are common features and may help discriminate from arterial ischaemia
3. Deep cerebral venous thrombosis often presents with depressed consciousness and diencephalic dysfunction but the clinical course may be much milder with symptoms such as hemiparesis
4. Investigations should include screening for the numerous inherited and acquired thrombophilic states associated with CVT
5. Anticoagulation with heparin followed by oral vitamin K antagonist is recommended and is not contraindicated by haemorrhagic venous infarct at the time of presentation

Key Radiological Learning Points
1. Imaging is used to detect the venous thrombosis itself, resultant venous ischaemia and complications such as haemorrhage and hydrocephalus
2. Acute intraluminal thrombus appears high attenuation on non-contrast CT
3. The MRI signal of venous thrombus evolves over time and distinguishing from flowing blood may be difficult, particularly in the first few days after clot formation and in the chronic stages
4. Venous infarcts are frequently haemorrhagic, bilateral and do not conform to arterial territories
5. Plain CT and MR should be supplemented by CT or MR venography when clinical suspicion is high

References

1. Leach JL, Fortuna RB, Jones BV, et al. Imaging of cerebral venous thrombosis: current techniques, spectrum of findings, and diagnostic pitfalls. Radiographics. 2006;26 Suppl 1: S19–41.
2. Saposnik G, Barinagarrementeria F, Brown RD Jr, et al. American Heart Association Stroke Council and the Council on Epidemiology and Prevention. Diagnosis and management of cerebral venous thrombosis: a statement for healthcare professionals from the American Heart Association/American Stroke Association. Stroke. 2011;42(4):1158–92.
3. Martinelli I, Passamonti SM, Rossi E, et al. Cerebral sinus-venous thrombosis. Intern Emerg Med. 2012;7 Suppl 3:S221–5.
4. Van den Bergh WM, van der Schaaf I, van Gijn J. The spectrum of presentations of venous infarction caused by deep cerebral vein thrombosis. Neurology. 2005;65(2):192–6.

5. Mullins ME, Grant PE, Wang B, et al. Parenchymal abnormalities associated with cerebral venous sinus thrombosis, assessment with diffusion weighted MR imaging. AJNR Am J Neuroradiol. 2004;25(10):1666–75.
6. Boukobza M, Crassard I, Bousser MG, et al. MR imaging features of isolated cortical vein thrombosis: diagnosis and follow up. AJNR Am J Neuroradiol. 2009;30(2):344–8.
7. Coutinho J, de Bruijn SFTM, deVeber G, et al. Anticoagulation for cerebral venous sinus thrombosis. Cochrane Database of Systematic Reviews. 2011, Issue 8. Art. No.: CD002005. doi:10.1002/14651858.CD002005.pub2.

Chapter 3
A Child with Enlarged Pupils

Georgios Niotakis and Vijeya Ganesan

Clinical History

A 3-year-old girl presented with recurrent episodes of transient unilateral limb and face weakness. Either side could be affected and initially the episodes resolved completely. Following an episode of persistent right hemiparesis, she was admitted to the local paediatric neurology unit. She has been noted to have fixed, dilated pupils from birth. No cause had been found and there was no impairment of visual function. At 4 months of age she presented with dyspnoea and failure to thrive, and was found to be in heart failure. A persistent ductus arteriosus (PDA) was successfully treated with ligation at 5 months of age. Her parents commented that she had exertional wheeze.

Examination

On examination, fixed dilated pupils were confirmed. She had mild bilateral ptosis, a rather immobile face, and long tract signs on the right with increased tone and brisk reflexes in the limbs. Cutaneous and cardiorespiratory examination were unremarkable.

G. Niotakis
Paediatric Neurology, Great Ormond Street Hospital for Children, London, UK

V. Ganesan, MRCPCH, MD (✉)
Neurosciences Unit, UCL Institute of Child Health, London, UK
e-mail: v.ganesan@ucl.ac.uk

© Springer-Verlag London 2015   17
S.K. Gill et al. (eds.), *Stroke Medicine: Case Studies from Queen Square*,
DOI 10.1007/978-1-4471-6705-1_3

Investigations

MRI showed an acute infarct in the border zone between the left MCA and ACA territories. There were gliotic scars in the white matter of both hemispheres, suggesting previous ischaemic injury in the deep border zones (Fig. 3.1). MRA showed bilateral intracranial occlusive arteriopathy. Cerebral angiography confirmed bilateral intracranial carotid occlusion with a number of angiographic features that were distinct from that seen in patients with moyamoya disease (Fig. 3.2). Echocardiography showed normal aortic calibre. Chest x-ray was normal.

Clinical Progress

The history of congenital mydriasis, PDA and respiratory symptoms led to the suspicion of an underlying systemic problem affecting smooth muscle, and specifically that her arteriopathy might be a consequence of a mutation in the *ACTA2* gene. She was subsequently shown to have an *R179H* mutation in this gene, confirming the diagnosis of occlusive cerebral arteriopathy associated with an *ACTA2* mutation.

She was treated with aspirin but continued to have TIAs, often many times a day. She showed only minimal recovery from the completed left hemisphere stroke. Her symptoms were thought to be haemodynamic in origin and she therefore underwent revascularisation surgery with encephaloarteriodurosynangiosis, initially to the right and then to the left hemisphere. In the immediate post-operative period, she experienced minor fluctuation of blood pressure (mean around 10 mmHg lower than baseline) but was not able to tolerate this and developed bilateral border zone infarcts. Subsequently, she had a residual pseudobulbar palsy

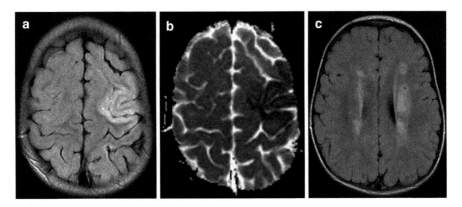

Fig. 3.1 (**a**) Axial T2-weighted (**b**) apparent diffusion coefficient map (**c**) axial FLAIR images at presentation. (**a**) and (**b**) show evidence of an acute infarct in the border zone between the left ACA and MCA territories. (**c**) shows signal change and cavitation in the deep white matter of both hemispheres indicating a combination of border zone and small vessel ischaemia

with significant speech and feeding difficulties as well as cognitive impairment. She had a spastic tetraparesis but was ambulant with aids. She has not had further strokes or TIAs.

Discussion

This case highlights two points about childhood stroke, which also applies to young adult stroke: (i) the evaluation of a young person with cerebrovascular disease should include consideration of a systemic or genetic diagnosis [1] and (ii) careful analysis of radiological phenotypes is important. In this case, the patient was initially given a diagnosis of moyamoya disease on the basis of the bilateral intracranial arteriopathy until the imaging was carefully reviewed.

ACTA2 codes for α-actin, the major contractile protein in smooth muscle cells (SMC). Mutations in *ACTA2* have been linked with diffuse and diverse vascular diseases, including thoracic aortic aneurysms and dissection (TAAD), and premature coronary and cerebrovascular disease [2]. Mutations disrupting R179 are associated with the most severe and multisystem phenotype, including cerebrovascular disease, bladder and gut problems [3]. All the cases described to date have congenital mydriasis and a history of PDA, important clinical clues [4].

The cerebral arteriopathy associated with *ACTA2* mutations was initially miscategorised as moyamoya disease. However, it has distinctive features from those seen in moyamoya disease (Fig. 3.2) [4]. In addition to the ischaemic brain injury, an

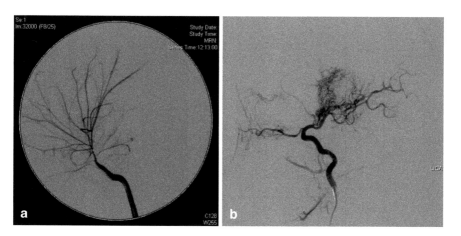

Fig. 3.2 Catheter cerebral angiogram, ICA injection, lateral projection in (**a**) the child described with an R179H mutation in *ACTA2* contrasted with (**b**) a child with idiopathic moyamoya disease. (**a**) Features of the *ACTA2* arteriopathy are the proximal ICA ectasia, terminal ICA narrowing, absence of basal "moyamoya" collaterals and the straight appearance of the intracranial arteries. In contrast, the patient in (**b**) has focal occlusion of the terminal ICA and the typical "puff of smoke" basal collaterals seen in moyamoya

additional radiological clue to this diagnosis is the presence of leukoaraiosis with signal change in the white matter, possibly representing small vessel involvement. This is a very unusual pattern in young children. We have anecdotally observed that these patients have a much higher incidence of perioperative complications related to revascularisation surgery than those with moyamoya disease. All cases to date have been *de novo* but other mutations in *ACTA2* show dominant inheritance. Affected individuals need regular screening for aortic dilatation and manifestations in other organ systems.

Key Clinical Learning Points
1. The evaluation of young people with complex cerebrovascular disease should involve consideration of a systemic or genetic cause
2. This should particularly focus on cutaneous (for neurocutaneous stigmata), cardiovascular examination as well as observation of dysmorphic features
3. *ACTA2* mutations lead to diffuse and diverse vascular diseases with multisystem manifestations including PDA, congenital mydriasis, pulmonary hypertension, gastrointestinal and bladder problems, as well as the cerebrovascular disease
4. Patients with occlusive arteriopathies may be very sensitive to even minor fluctuations in systemic blood pressure

Key Radiological Learning Points
1. Critical analysis of imaging is crucial to identifying novel phenotypes and differentiating between diagnostic entities; intracranial occlusive arteriopathies in young people are not all moyamoya disease
2. The key features that differentiate *ACTA2* ateriopathy from moyamoya disease are (i) proximal ICA ectasia (ii) distal ICA occlusive disease (iii) no basal collaterals (iv) straight intracranial arteries (v) leukoariotic signal change in white matter

References

1. Munot P, Crow YJ, Ganesan V. Paediatric stroke: genetic insights into disease mechanisms and treatment targets. Lancet Neurol. 2011;10(3):264–74.
2. Guo DC, Papke CL, Tran-Fadulu V, et al. Mutations in smooth muscle alpha-actin (ACTA2) cause coronary artery disease, stroke, and moyamoya disease, along with thoracic aortic disease. Am J Hum Genet. 2009;84(5):617–27.

3. Milewicz DM, Østergaard JR, Ala-Kokko LM, et al. De novo ACTA2 mutation causes a novel syndrome of multisystemic smooth muscle dysfunction. Am J Med Genet A. 2010;152A(10):2437–43.
4. Munot P, Saunders DE, Milewicz DM, et al. A novel distinctive cerebrovascular phenotype is associated with heterozygous Arg179 ACTA2 mutations. Brain. 2012;135(Pt 8):2506–14.

Chapter 4
Locked in or Break Out?

Fiona Kennedy

Clinical History

A 61-year-old woman was admitted to the Accident and Emergency department. Less than 3 hours earlier, she developed sudden onset aphasia and weakness of her right upper limb and the right side of her face. Earlier that day, around 12.30 pm, she complained of dizziness, vertigo and nausea of sudden onset. She visited her GP at 6 pm when it was discovered that she was in atrial fibrillation (AF). She had a past medical history of hypertension, hypercholesterolaemia, deep vein thrombosis and type 2 diabetes mellitus.

Examination

On examination, her blood pressure was 149/80 mmHg and the heart rate was 118 beats/min with an irregularly irregular rhythm. Electrocardiogram (ECG) confirmed atrial fibrillation. On neurological examination, she appeared aphasic and had a left gaze palsy. The pupils were equal and reacting to light. Both left lower limb and right upper limb demonstrated a flexor response to painful stimulation. The tendon reflexes were brisk in the right upper limb. There was hypertonia in both lower limbs with bilateral extensor plantar responses. Her National Institute of Health Stroke Score (NIHSS) was 24 with a Glasgow Coma Score (GCS) of 10/15 (E4, M4, V2).

Shortly after arriving at hospital, her GCS dropped to 7. Examination revealed that she had developed an incomplete locked-in syndrome.

F. Kennedy, MB, Bch, BAO, MRCP (UK)
Stroke Research Group, Department of Brain Repair and Rehabilitation, UCL Institute
of Neurology, University College London, National Hospital for Neurology
and Neurosurgery, London, UK
e-mail: fiona.kennedy@ucl.ac.uk

© Springer-Verlag London 2015
S.K. Gill et al. (eds.), *Stroke Medicine: Case Studies from Queen Square*,
DOI 10.1007/978-1-4471-6705-1_4

Investigations

CT revealed an occlusive thrombus in the distal basilar artery and possibly low attenuation in the right mid brain/pons (Figs. 4.1 and 4.2). The right vertebral artery was of tiny calibre throughout its length and was difficult to identify beyond V2 (approximately the level of 6th cervical vertebrae). The radiologist commented that the latter finding might be explained by occlusion or stenosis, but might also be a normal congenital variant. As a consequence of the patient's presentation, deterioration and the CT findings, she was transferred to the Intensive Therapy Unit (ITU). Despite being 10 hours from the onset of initial symptoms, it was decided to administer intravenous thrombolysis because her level of consciousness and clinical state had deteriorated in the last 3 hours.

Clinical Progress

It was concluded that she had basilar artery thrombosis causing mid-pontine infarction and locked-in syndrome. Her imaging was discussed at the neurovascular multidisciplinary meeting and the consensus opinion was that the narrow vertebral artery was a congenital variant and that new-onset AF had been the source of an

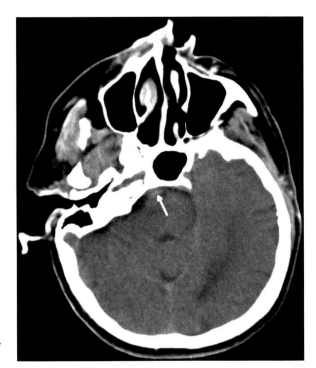

Fig. 4.1 Unenhanced CT image showing hyperdense thrombus in prepontine basilar artery (*white arrow*) with subtle pontine low density in keeping with early ischaemic change

Fig. 4.2 Unenhanced CT image from another patient showing the typical hyperdense basilar artery sign. Note the density of the basilar artery (*solid white arrow*) is higher than visualised segment of right terminal internal carotid artery (*dashed white arrow*)

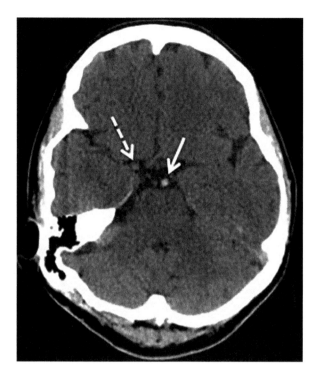

embolus to the basilar artery, which had then propagated to cause progression of her symptoms.

She was commenced on warfarin for secondary prevention as well as antihypertensive medication and a statin. She remained on the ITU for almost one month. A per-endoscopic gastrostomy (PEG) tube was inserted to improve nutrition because of poor swallow and risk of aspiration. Follow up CT showed bilateral pontine and superior left cerebellar hemispheric low attenuation consistent with established infarction, explaining the crossed signs on examination. MRI showed extensive recent infarction surrounding the ponto-medullary junction, but by the time of the MRI, the basilar artery was patent.

The patient was transferred from ITU to the acute stroke unit, where she received intensive rehabilitation. She slowly improved and reached the level of communicating via head nodding and lip reading before being transferred to her local hospital to continue rehabilitation. She was eventually discharged home 5 months after stroke onset.

Discussion

Basilar artery thrombosis is an uncommon cause of stroke but it is associated with a very poor prognosis [1, 2]. The mortality rate associated with basilar artery thrombosis has been reported as high as 90% [3], but with modern intensive management

Table 4.1 The possible
presenting symptoms and
signs of a patient with basilar
syndrome

Symptoms and signs
Drowsiness
Coma
Dizziness
Ataxia
Confusion
Headache
Hemiparesis
Hemisensory disturbance
Locked-in syndrome
Oculomotor palsies
Nystagmus
Facial palsy
Oropharyngeal palsy
Crossed-signs
Homonymous hemianopia
Cortical blindness

the early mortality rate is much lower. The most common causes of basilar occlusion are local atherosclerosis in the basilar artery, occlusion due to an embolism from cardiac or large artery sources, spontaneous or traumatic arterial dissection, fusiform aneurysms, meningitis, arteritis, and complications of endovascular or neurosurgical procedures [1, 2]. In this case, the basilar artery thrombosis was caused by an embolism from the heart. Although commonly presenting in middle age, basilar thrombosis can present at any age, including in children [4].

The clinical presentation and prognosis of stroke secondary to basilar artery disease varies depending on the level of the stenosis or occlusion. More than 60% of patients give a history of preceding symptoms of transient ischaemia in the vertebrobasilar territory [1, 5, 6], including vertigo and nausea, headache, diplopia, dysarthria, homonymous hemianopia or cortical blindness, hemiparesis and hemisensory disturbance. The majority of patients then go on to have a posterior circulation stroke. On the other hand, there are a proportion of patients who do not have any prodromal symptoms but rather present with an established infarct. Sudden embolic or thrombotic occlusions can cause extensive ischaemic damage and severe clinical deficits [1]. Large pontine infarction results from occlusion of the proximal or middle basilar segments and presents with hemi- or quadriplegia, reduced consciousness, dysarthria, dysphagia, oculomotor and cranial nerve palsies. Occlusion of the distal basilar can cause stroke bilaterally in the mesencephalon and thalami leading to a reduced conscious level, quadriparesis, nuclear and supranuclear gaze palsies. Patients can present as confused and amnesic when the thalami are involved. Occlusion extending into the posterior cerebral artery territory will result in hemianopia or cortical blindness [1]. Similarly, when the temporal or occipital lobes are affected on one or both sides, patients present with visual and oculomotor symptoms as well as behavioural abnormalities including somnolence, agitation and hallucinations (Table 4.1). The location of thrombosis can also be used to predict the prognosis; distal basilar occlusion has been shown to have a higher survival rate compared with thrombus in the middle or proximal portion of the artery [4].

The 'locked-in' syndrome occurs with large pontine infarction and patients present with quadriplegia, bilateral facial weakness, anarthria and aphagia. Horizontal gaze palsy may also be evident, leaving only vertical eye movement and eye blinking intact. Patients are awake and alert but their only form of communication may be via blinking of the eyes [1]. This may lead to the inexperienced misdiagnosing aphasia (as in this case), unconsciousness, or even functional illness.

This case demonstrates many of the clinical dilemmas associated with basilar artery thrombosis and posterior circulation stroke. When a patient presents with symptoms suggestive of posterior circulation thrombosis it is imperative to have a high index of suspicion and act fast in the face of a grave prognosis. Treatment of posterior circulation thrombosis is based on evidence from small case-series or single case reports [5–18]. There are no current randomised controlled trials (RCTs) published that evaluate the efficacy of intravenous or intra-arterial thrombolysis or endovascular treatment such as mechanical clot retrieval. Even published RCTs of thrombolysis in acute stroke have not included many patients with posterior circulation stroke. There are many renowned trials that demonstrate the efficacy and safety of treatment for carotid artery stenosis but such evidence does not yet exist for the vertebrobasilar circulation. Despite the void of evidence from controlled trials in this area, the reports that exist suggest a trend towards treating these patients with thrombolysis or endovascular clot extraction to improve their clinical and functional outcome. However, it is clear that patients who commence treatment with antithrombotic agents of any type while they have only moderately disabling signs have a better outcome than those that are only treated when they are already locked-in [19].

Observational studies and case reports have been published which have investigated the use of antithrombotics (AT), thrombolysis and endovascular treatment in basilar thrombosis [7, 22]. The key to a better survival rate and functional outcome is recanalization. In one study of 50 consecutive patients, 46% of patients in whom recanalization with IVT was achieved were independent at 3 months [7]. In the same study none of the patients with failed recanalization were independent at 3 months. In other studies a higher rate of recanalization has been achieved with intra-arterial thrombolysis [23]. Despite these important results some patients do not recanalize successfully with thrombolysis and as expected the outcome for these patients is much worse.

In 2004 a systematic analysis was published comparing treatment of basilar artery thrombosis with intravenous thrombolysis and intra-arterial thrombolysis (IAT) [24]. This analysis highlighted the poor prognosis of basilar thrombosis with equal rates of death and dependency in each treatment group. Survival rates, percentage of good outcomes and frequency of complications were the same in both groups. Recanalization was achieved more frequently in the group of patients treated with IAT (65% versus 58%, p = 0.05). Like the other studies published, this analysis concluded that the likelihood of a good outcome without recanalization was "close to nil".

As well as thrombolysis, there has been a recent trend towards treating basilar thrombosis endovascularly. These techniques include clot aspiration, angioplasty and stenting, laser treatment, ultrasound, and clot retrieval [20, 21, 25–28]. The Basilar Artery International Cooperation Study (BASICS) was a prospective observational study of 592 patients with radiologically confirmed basilar artery occlusion [19]. In this study the patients were divided into three groups according to the treatment they received; antithrombotic therapy alone (AT), primary intravenous thrombolysis (IVT) including subsequent IA thrombolysis, or intra-arterial therapy (IAT) which included thrombolysis, mechanical clot retrieval, stenting or a combination of these treatments. BASICS did not show any superiority of one treatment over the other, however, consistent with other published data, BASICS showed that recanalization did protect against poorer outcome.

As with thrombolysis treatment of any stroke, patients treated by endovascular techniques are at risk of complications for example intracerebral haemorrhage, perforation of cerebral vessels, subarachnoid haemorrhage, haemorrhagic transformation and extracranial haemorrhage. These complications plus failed recanalization contribute to the high mortality and morbidity association with basilar thrombosis.

Several groups have completed work looking at prognostic factors that may influence the outcome of treatment which include time from onset to presentation, baseline mRs and NIHSS, degree of ischaemic damage on baseline neuroimaging and evidence of sufficient collateral circulation on angiogram. Currently the evidence shows a non-significant trend for favourable outcome in patients who are treated within 6 hours, in patients who have a low baseline NIHSS, patients with sufficient collaterals and patients with little ischaemic damage on baseline imaging [23]. However, not all studies come to the same conclusion. One showed an increase complication rate of haemorrhagic transformation in patients treated within 10 hours of onset [29]. Our patient was treated with thrombolysis at approximately 10 hours after symptom onset, she had a baseline NIHSS of 24, and there was evidence of subacute infarction in the posterior fossa on baseline CT, yet despite these poor prognostic factors she was treated successfully. This highlights the importance of making management decisions on an individual patient basis.

There is an argument for extending the time window for thrombolysis in patients with basilar artery thrombosis because of the poor prognosis associated with treating these patients conservatively. Extending the time to treatment in this cohort of patients may incur benefit on some of the patients. A study by Cross et al. published in 1997 did not show any increase in thrombolysis-related complications in patients who were treated after 10 hours compared to those patients treated within 10 hours [29].

In conclusion, despite the lack of evidence from randomised controlled trials, the diagnosis and treatment of patients who present with basilar thrombosis should be fast and effective. Evidence does not suggest superiority of one treatment over the other, but the message from published studies is that recanalization is associated with a better outcome in most cases and that basilar artery occlusion is a treatable condition, and no longer always the fatal dismal diagnosis it was in the past.

> **Key Clinical Learning Points**
> 1. Basilar occlusion is associated with a grave prognosis if not treated promptly
> 2. There is a lack of randomised evidence to suggest the best way to manage patients presenting with basilar occlusion
> 3. Treatment options currently include antithrombotics, intravenous or intra-arterial thrombolysis, and mechanical clot retrieval
> 4. Recanalization is associated with a better prognosis
> 5. Management decisions should be made on an individual patient basis with multi-disciplinary team input

References

1. Mattle HP, Arnold M, Lindsberg PJ, et al. Basilar artery occlusion. Lancet Neurol. 2011;10:1002–14.
2. Voetsch B, DeWitt D, Pessin MS, et al. Basilar artery occlusive disease in the New England Medical Centre Posterior Circulation Registry. Arch Neurol. 2004;61:496–504.
3. Baird TA, Muir KW, Bone I. Basilar artery occlusion. Neurocrit Care. 2004;1:319–30.
4. Richardson PG. Basilar artery thrombosis. Emerg Med. 2001;13:367–72.
5. Archer CR, Horenstein S. Basilar artery occlusion: clinical and radiographic correlation. Stroke. 1977;8:383–91.
6. Ferbert A, Bruckman H, Drunmen R. Clinical features of proven basilar artery occlusion. Stroke. 1990;21:1135–42.
7. Lindsberg PJ, Soinne L, Tatlisumak T, et al. Long-term outcome after intravenous thrombolysis of basilar artery occlusion. JAMA. 2004;292:1862–6.
8. Brandt T, von Kummer R, Muller-Kuppers M, et al. Thrombolytic therapy of acute basilar artery occlusion: variables affecting recanalization and outcome. Stroke. 1996;27:875–81.
9. Bergui M, Stura G, Daniele D, et al. Mechanical thrombolysis in ischaemic stroke attributable to basilar artery occlusion as first-line treatment. Stroke. 2006;37:145–50.
10. Wang H, Foster K, Wang D, et al. Successful intra-arterial basilar artery thrombolysis in a patient with bilateral vertebral artery occlusion; technical case report. Neurosurgery. 2005;57 suppl 4:e398.
11. Wijdicks EFM, Nichols DA, Thielen KR, et al. Intra-arterial thrombolysis in acute basilar artery thromboembolism: the initial Mayo Clinic experience. Mayo Clin Proc. 1997;72:1005–13.
12. Jung S, Mono ML, Fischer U, et al. Three-month and long-term outcomes and their predictors in acute basilar artery occlusion treated with intra-arterial thrombolysis. Stroke. 2011;42:1946–51.
13. Hacke W, Zeumer H, Ferbert A, et al. Intra-arterial thrombolytic therapy improves outcome in patients with acute vertebrobasilar occlusive disease. Stroke. 1988;19:1216–22.
14. Macleod MR, David SM, Mitchell PJ, et al. Results of a multicentre, randomised controlled trial of intra-arterial urokinase in the treatment of acute posterior circulation ischaemic stroke. Cerebrovasc Dis. 2005;20(1):12–7.
15. Lin DDM, Gailloud P, Beauchamp NJ, et al. Combined stent placement and thrombolysis in acute vertebrobasilar ischaemic stroke. AJNR Am J Neuroradiol. 2003;24:1827–33.

16. Chapot R, Houdart E, Rogopoulos A, et al. Thromboaspiration in the basilar artery: report of two cases. AJNR Am J Neuroradiol. 2002;23:282–4.
17. Mordasini P, Brekenfeld C, Byrne JV, et al. Technical feasibility and application of mechanical thrombectomy with the Solitaire FR revascularization device in acute basilar artery occlusion. AJNR Am J Neuroradiol. 2013;34(1):159–63. doi:10.3174/ajnr.A3168.
18. Gress DR, Smith WS, Dowd CF, et al. Angioplasty for intracranial symptomatic vertebrobasilar ischaemia. Neurosurgery. 2002;51:23–9.
19. Schonewille WJ, Wijman CAC, Michel P, et al. on behalf of the BASICS Study Group. Treatment and outcomes of acute basilar artery occlusion in the Basilar Artery International Cooperation Study (BASICS): a prospective registry study. Lancet Neurol. 2009;8:724–30.
20. Mayer TE, Hamann GF, Brueckman HJ. Treatment of basilar artery embolism with a mechanical extraction device: necessity of flow reversal. Stroke. 2002;33:2232–5.
21. Zaidat OO, Tolbert M, Smith TP, et al. Primary endovascular therapy with clot retrieval and balloon angioplasty for acute basilar artery occlusion. Pediatr Neurosurg. 2005;41:323–7.
22. Yu W, Binder D, Foster-Barber A, et al. Endovascular embolectomy of acute basilar artery occlusion. Neurology. 2003;61:1421–3.
23. Arnold M, Nedeltchev K, Schroth G, et al. Clinical and radiological predictors of recanalization and outcome of 40 patients with acute basilar artery occlusion treated with intra-arterial thrombolysis. J Neurol Neurosurg Psychiatry. 2004;75:857–62.
24. Lindsberg PJ, Mattle HP. Therapy of basilar artery occlusion: a systematic analysis comparing intra-arterial and intravenous thrombolysis. Stroke. 2006;37:922–8.
25. Gobin YP, Starkman S, Duckwiler GR, et al. MERCI I: a phase 1 study of mechanical embolus removal in cerebral ischaemia. Stroke. 2004;35:2848–54.
26. Leary MC, Saver JL, Gobin YP, et al. Beyond tissue plasminogen activator: mechanical intervention in acute stroke. Ann Emerg Med. 2003;41:838–46.
27. Kerber CW, Barr JD, Berger RM, et al. Snare retrieval of intracranial thrombus in patients with acute stroke. J Vasc Interv Radiol. 2002;13:1269–74.
28. Nedeltchev K, Remonda L, Do DD, et al. Acute stenting and thromboaspiration in basilar artery occlusions due to embolism from the dominating vertebral artery. Neuroradiology. 2004;46:686–91.
29. Cross III DT, Moran CJ, Akins PT, et al. Relationship between clot location and outcome after basilar artery thrombolysis. AJNR Am J Neuroradiol. 1997;18:1221–8.

Chapter 5
An Unusual TIA

David Doig and Fiona Kennedy

Clinical History

A 54-year-old retired printer presented to hospital with an isolated tonic-clonic seizure of around 5 min duration followed by an episode of post-ictal confusion. He had been attending an outpatient clinic at the hospital with a 3-year history of attacks of weakness affecting the right arm and leg, occurring once each month or more frequently. These attacks resulted in collapse, which the patient described as his "legs giving way", and which was sometimes preceded by a pre-syncopal feeling of dizziness or light-headedness. The weakness completely resolved within a minute on each occasion. There was no loss of consciousness associated with these episodes, no visual symptoms and no sensory disturbance. Speech was unaffected. His father had noticed considerable decline in his son's cognitive functioning over several years. The patient himself was not aware of any problems with his memory.

This patient smoked cigarettes and had prior diagnoses of hypertension and hypercholesterolaemia. There was uncertainty as to whether his GP had also previously diagnosed diabetes. There was a past history of alcohol excess, with consumption of up to two bottles of wine per day, and a positive family history of vascular disease.

D. Doig, MBChB, BScMedSci (Hons), MRCP (✉)
F. Kennedy, MB, Bch, BAO, MRCP (UK)
Stroke Research Group, Department of Brain Repair and Rehabilitation, UCL Institute of Neurology, University College London, National Hospital for Neurology and Neurosurgery, London, UK
e-mail: d.doig@ucl.ac.uk; fiona.kennedy@ucl.ac.uk

© Springer-Verlag London 2015
S.K. Gill et al. (eds.), *Stroke Medicine: Case Studies from Queen Square*,
DOI 10.1007/978-1-4471-6705-1_5

Examination

After recovery from the seizure, examination of the central nervous system was unremarkable apart from some generally brisk reflexes. Of note there was no limb weakness on examination of the peripheral nervous system, and no speech disturbance. The patient was orientated in time and date, but was not able to give the name or location of the hospital.

Neuropsychological testing revealed marked cognitive decline for his age group relative to an estimated low average/average predicted pre-morbid estimated ability. In particular, there was impairment of executive function and speed of information processing. Symptoms of low mood and anxiety were reported, but these were not sufficient to explain the psychometric findings.

Radiological Investigations

MRI brain showed infarction in the anterior and posterior border zones of the left MCA territory. Comparison with previous imaging revealed that the volume of infarction had increased on serial scans since his first clinic attendances. Mature infarcts were also present in the left frontal and occipital lobes, and to a lesser extent in the left parietal lobe. This was thought to account for at least part of his cognitive decline.

Carotid duplex ultrasound reported absent flow in the left ICA. CTA and MRA confirmed complete occlusion of the left ICA (Fig. 5.1), but also demonstrated right ICA stenosis and a tight stenosis of the left VA origin.

Catheter angiography was performed and confirmed the occlusion of the left ICA. The vertebrobasilar system was shown to provide perfusion to the left MCA territory via a patent posterior communicating artery (PoCA). There was no flow across the anterior communicating artery to the left hemisphere. A "shelf-like" 60% stenosis of the right ICA and severe stenosis of the left VA were confirmed. CT perfusion demonstrated significantly delayed transit time and reduced cerebral blood flow in the cortical territories of the left MCA territory with marked reduction in perfusion in the anterior and posterior border zones of the left MCA (Fig. 5.2).

A diagnosis of chronic hypoperfusion of the left cerebral hemisphere with resultant left MCA territory border zone infarction was made.

Clinical Progress

The patient was already taking a statin, ramipril, aspirin and dipyridamole. After discussion between the patient, his family, and a multi-disciplinary team of neurologists, surgeons and interventional neuroradiologists, a left vertebral stent

Fig. 5.1 Reconstructed image from MR angiogram demonstrating occlusion of the left ICA above the carotid bifurcation (*arrowed*)

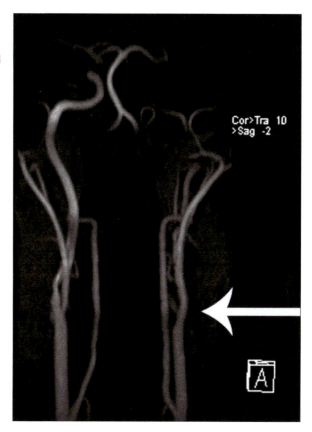

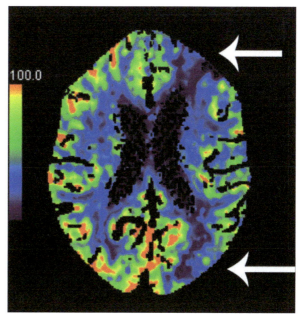

Fig. 5.2 Representative slice from CT perfusion colour map demonstrating reduced perfusion of left MCA/ACA and MCA/PCA borderzone territories (*arrowed*). The scale shows cerebral blood flow in ml/min/100 g brain tissue; yellow and red colours indicate higher flow and purple and blue colours lower flow

was inserted across the VA stenosis to improve perfusion to the left MCA through the patent PCA. The lack of flow to the left hemisphere from the right carotid was thought to render right carotid endarterectomy futile in this setting.

Discussion

The main mechanism by which carotid atherosclerosis becomes symptomatic is plaque rupture and thromboembolism. However, this patient presented with an occluded carotid artery and symptoms attributable to cerebral hypoperfusion. Haemodynamic impairment is an under-recognized cause of cerebral or retinal stroke or TIA, and series of consecutive cases estimate that this may be the underlying mechanism in up to 10% of patients [1].

Haemodynamic impairment of the supply to one hemisphere of the brain may cause focal neurological deficit akin to TIA or stroke. However, episodes may be stereotyped and frequent – features which are uncommon in embolic disease. Clues in the history to suggest hypoperfusion include symptoms inducible by changes in neck positioning or postural change, coughing or Valsalva manoeuvre, or the association between low blood pressure and the onset of symptoms perhaps due to postural hypotension or occurring after meals as a result of diversion of blood flow to the gut. There may be a history of "limb-shaking" TIA, which can be mistaken for focal seizure. These episodes are characterized by rhythmic shaking of the arm and/or leg, which may be accompanied by weakness on the affected side [2]. However, in haemodynamic TIA, there is usually no march of symptoms or impairment of consciousness more typical of epilepsy, EEG studies of symptomatic patients show no epileptiform activity and anticonvulsants are generally ineffective [3]. A proposed pathophysiological mechanism for generation of these symptoms is primary hyperexcitability of ischaemic neurons, or alternatively a loss of normal inhibitory pathways [4]. In the eye, inducible hypoperfusion of the retina, which is supplied by the ophthalmic artery arising from the internal carotid, may be reported as "whiteout" of vision in one eye when exposed to bright light.

Carotid occlusion is associated with an increased risk of delayed ipsilateral stroke. Identified risk factors for stroke in this context include cerebral (rather than retinal) symptoms, the presence of limb-shaking TIA and the presence of leptomeningeal collaterals. Asymptomatic patients with carotid occlusion may be at lower risk [5].

Carotid occlusion is most reliably detected using non-invasive angiography by CTA. MRA and carotid duplex ultrasound may misinterpret as occluded a carotid artery that is still patent, when the artery is collapsed with very low flow ("trickle flow" or "pseudo-occlusion"). Ultrasound also has the disadvantage of showing only a short segment of the ICA and more distal occlusion may not be seen. Catheter angiography may be required to confirm the diagnosis. The small risk of stroke during catheter angiography is justified if revascularisation is being considered. Selective angiography has the addition advantage of showing which cerebral arterial territories are supplied by each carotid or vertebral artery.

CT or MR perfusion, or single-photon emission computed tomography (SPECT), are valuable in confirming areas of reduced cerebral blood flow, while trans-cranial Doppler ultrasound (TCD) may be used to demonstrate the direction of flow in individual branches of the Circle of Willis and the MCA supply from collateral vessels [6].

Structural brain MRI is also important in diagnosis of haemodynamic infarction, and in addition to the patterns of wedge-shaped border zone infarction seen in this case, often reveals infarction in the deep white matter border zones in the centrum semiovale in a "rosary" or "string of beads" pattern [7]. Occasionally, this pattern of infarction is found in a patient with only a mild stenosis or even a widely patent ICA, which suggests that the ICA may have been temporarily occluded at the time of symptoms by thrombus which then lysed rapidly. Bilateral border zone infarction may be seen after an episode of cardiac arrest or severely reduced cardiac output compromising flow to both hemispheres.

Patients with carotid occlusion have significant vascular disease, and therefore control of vascular risk factors is essential. Cautious blood pressure control, avoiding hypotension, antithrombotic drugs and management of cholesterol are all advised [5]. Some authors advocate increasing blood pressure if symptoms are persistent and occur in settings where hypotension is a likely cause. However, this strategy alone may not be enough to eliminate symptoms and carries a significant risk of promoting stroke. Therefore we do not advocate this policy.

Revascularisation strategies to prevent haemodynamic stroke are controversial. The STA-MCA Bypass Study [8] and Carotid Occlusion Surgery Study [9] have both studied the procedure of EC-IC bypass (in which an extracranial vessel such as the superficial temporal artery is surgically anastomosed to a segment of the middle cerebral artery to restore perfusion pressure) in the setting of ipsilateral carotid occlusion. Although good graft patency, improved perfusion of the affected territory and elimination of clinical symptoms are possible, this is at the expense of a high perioperative stroke rate of up to 15%, and there does not appear to be a reduction in the overall rate of ipsilateral stroke in the long term. We therefore advocate surgery or stenting to improve collateral supply in the contralateral ICA or the VA if these are significantly stenosed (>50%).

Key Clinical Learning Points
1. Hypoperfusion is an under-recognized mechanism of cerebral and retinal ischaemia and infarction secondary to critical carotid ICA stenosis or occlusion
2. The diagnosis is made through careful history and examination with appropriate angiography and cerebral perfusion studies
3. Management of vascular risk factors is essential but may not abolish symptoms
4. EC-IC bypass surgery may alleviate symptoms but is not proven to reduce the medium- or long-term rate of recurrent stroke
5. Revascularisation of the contralateral ICA of VA stenosis may be beneficial

Key Radiological Learning Points
1. Parenchymal imaging in patients in whom haemodynamic mechanisms have caused or contributed to symptoms shows characteristic location of infarction in the superficial cortical and deep border zones
2. Occlusion may be misdiagnosed on non-invasive MRA and carotid duplex ultrasound. Catheter angiogram may be required to confirm the diagnosis and additionally demonstrate which artery is perfusing the territory of the occluded artery
3. Perfusion imaging is useful in demonstrating reduced cerebral blood flow in the affected territory

References

1. Bladin CF, Chambers BR. Frequency and pathogenesis of haemodynamic stroke. Stroke. 1994;25:2179–81.
2. Ali S, Khan MA, Khealani B. Limb-shaking transient ischemic attacks: case report and review of literature. BMC Neurol. 2006;6:5.
3. Schultz UGR, Rothwell PM. Transient ischaemic attacks mimicking focal motor seizures. Postgrad Med J. 2002;78:246–7.
4. Han SW, Kim SH, Kim JK, et al. Haemodynamic changes in limb shaking TIA associated with anterior cerebral artery stenosis. Neurology. 2004;63:1519–21.
5. Persoon S, Kappelle LJ, Klijn CJM. Limb-shaking transient ischaemic attacks in patients with internal carotid artery occlusion: a case–control study. Brain. 2010;113:915–22.
6. Vernieri F, Tibuzzi F, Pasqualetti P, et al. Transcranial Doppler and near-infrared spectroscopy can evaluate the haemodynamic effect of carotid artery occlusion. Stroke. 2004;35:64–72.
7. Klijn CJM, Kappelle LJ. Haemodynamic stroke: clinical features, prognosis and management. Lancet Neurol. 2010;9:1008–17.
8. Jefree RL, Stoodley MA. STA-MCA bypass for symptomatic carotid occlusion and haemodynamic impairment. J Clin Neurosci. 2009;16:226–35.
9. Kleiser B, Widder B. Course of carotid artery occlusions with impaired cerebrovascular reactivity. Stroke. 1992;23:171–4.

Chapter 6
Hemianopic Alexia

Ashvini Keshavan and Alexander Leff

Clinical History

A 46-year-old man was referred to the Queen Square hemianopia and higher visual functions clinic 4 years after his stroke. His main problem was slow and effortful reading.

A month prior to his stroke, he had cystoscopic ureteric dilatation following several months of colicky right flank pain without frank haematuria or dysuria. Three years previously he had renal calculi which passed spontaneously. The ureteroscopy showed a benign stricture in the context of a kink in the right ureter, without any obvious calculi. This was dilated using a balloon technique and no stent was placed, but he was offered an elective renal angiogram to rule out a vascular cause for this anatomical appearance.

The subsequent renal angiogram was a long procedure during which he began to experience agitation, low back pain and a mounting severe headache with blurred vision, disorientation and vomiting. His cardio-respiratory observations during the procedure were normal. He was transferred to an inpatient ward due to the persistence of his symptoms. Initially these were put down to migraine; however, his headache failed to settle and he described concomitant visual blurring, nausea, inability to stand and problems with short-term memory. On examination he had impaired short-term recall, a right homonymous hemianopia, distal right leg weakness and numbness in the sole of his foot. He was also completely unable to read.

A. Keshavan, MB, BChir
Department of Neurology, Department of Brain Repair and Rehabilitation,
UCL Institute of Neurology, University College London and National Hospital for Neurology and Neurosurgery, London, UK

A. Leff, PhD, FRCP (✉)
Institute of Cognitive Neuroscience and Department of Brain Repair and Rehabilitation,
UCL Institute of Neurology, University College London and National Hospital for Neurology and Neurosurgery, London, UK
e-mail: a.leff@ucl.ac.uk

© Springer-Verlag London 2015
S.K. Gill et al. (eds.), *Stroke Medicine: Case Studies from Queen Square*,
DOI 10.1007/978-1-4471-6705-1_6

An MRI brain scan was requested. This showed widespread oedema in the left cerebral hemisphere. His short-term memory recovered within 10 weeks, and he regained full power in his right leg although he had some residual numbness in the ball of the right foot. The following investigations were normal: MRA, a transthoracic echocardiogram and a 24-hour tape recording of his ECG. The likeliest cause was thought to be thrombo-embolism to the left cerebral hemisphere related to his angiogram.

He managed a structured return to office work after 7 months, and his reading improved such that he could name letters and manage most words easily; but even 4 years after the initial event, he continued to have difficulty in reading; he was accurate but slow. He did not have symptoms affecting any other language functions; for example, speech production, speech perception and writing were all normal. He was able to recognise faces and navigate normally apart from occasionally bumping into things on his right-hand side. His work as a business manager demanded many hours of reading text on computers and writing long documents. He had stopped driving because of his visual field defect.

There was no other past medical history or family history of note. He was taking aspirin 75 mg once daily on the recommendation of his stroke physician. He lived with his daughter and wife who was a special needs teacher. She helped him in the initial months after the stroke by suggesting a phonemics programme usually employed in teaching children with dyslexia. He found this helpful, and was keen to try any new method to improve his reading.

Examination

Bilateral visual acuity was 6/6 corrected with spectacles. He had a clear right-sided homonymous hemianopia with between 2° and 3° of sparing to the right of fixation. He could read single letters, but made one error in mistaking an [i] for an "l" and then thinking it might have been the number "one". He read words normally but took more time on longer words. He correctly identified real words and non-words from a list of these. On reading text, he managed 66 words per minute but with four errors. Three of these were self-corrected and all the errors occur at the end of the word (this is commonly seen in hemianopic alexia). For example, he misread [cause] as "causes" and [suggests] as "suggest". In summary he had evidence of a peripheral alexia with sparing of central language functions (alexia without agraphia). The history suggests that he suffered from global alexia initially (could not easily recognize letters), recovering through pure alexia (problems mainly at the word level) to his current situation, hemianopic alexia, where text reading problems predominate in the face of near-normal single word reading.

Investigations

A scan from 2010, 5 years post-stroke is shown (Fig. 6.1).

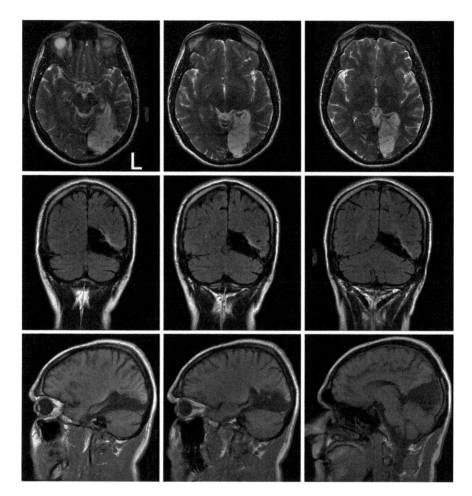

Fig. 6.1 MRI brain with: axial T2 sequence (*top row*, infarction is white); coronal FLAIR (*middle row*, infarction is black); and, sagittal T1 (*bottom row*, infarction is black). The medial occipital lobe has been affected including the calcarine cortex and its connections. Damage extends ventrally and laterally into occipito-temporal cortex with parts of the lingual gyrus, medial occipito-temporal sulcus (collateral sulcus) and medial fusiform gyrus all affected. The lateral portion of the fusiform gyrus and the corpus callosum are both spared

Neurological Rehabilitation

The patient's main symptom was his reduced reading speed, which was affecting both his work and leisure activities, so rehabilitation efforts were focussed on this. Reading laterally animated text that scrolls from right-to-left induces small-field optokinetic nystagmus and, with enough practice, this increases hemianopic alexic patients' text reading speed when they go back to static text [1, 2]. Read-Right is a free-to-use web-based application that includes tests of text reading and visual field estimation, as well as the therapy itself (laterally scrolling text): http://www.readright.ucl.ac.uk.

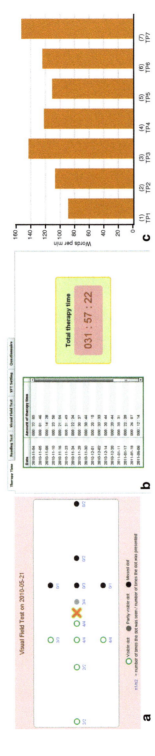

Fig. 6.2 All data was recorded on a secure server at UCL that hosts Read-Right. (**a**) Visual field test. This is taken binocularly with multiple points in the visual field tested in different combinations (see: http://www.readright.ucl.ac.uk/help/h_vid_vft.php for a video demonstration). The focus is on the horizontal meridian (as this is most important for reading) with points at 1°, 2.5°, 5° and 10° tested. He had a clear right-sided homonymous hemianopia with some macular sparing. (**b**) Total therapy time with dates. We suggest patients practice for roughly 20 min a day. (**c**) Therapy effects. Every time 5 hours of therapy are completed, the patient is prompted to test their text reading speed on a standardized test. He improved from baseline, 89 words per minute (wpm) [TP1], to 153 wpm 6 months later [TP7]. *TP* time point

We directed the patient to use the site where he estimated his visual fields (Fig. 6.2a), and practiced with the scrolling text for nearly 32 hours over a 6-month period (Fig. 6.2b). This lead to an improvement of his reading speeds by about 70% (Fig. 6.2c).

Discussion

Unlike many other impairments caused by stroke, homonymous visual field loss rarely improves after 6 months [3]. Despite this, patients can continue to make functional gains by utilizing their remaining vision by making more efficient eye movements [4]. Recent evidence suggest that eye movement therapy is task specific, so practicing making eye movements that improve visual search will not have a beneficial effect on reading eye movements and vice-versa [5].

Hemianopic alexia is the most common of the peripheral alexias and generally the least severe, although it has a big impact on most patients' lives [6]. Readers of texts written from left-to-right have particular problems when they have a right-sided homonymous hemianopia; they have difficulty with generating efficient reading eye movements because they are robbed of visual information about up-coming words. This effectively 'disconnects' the otherwise intact oculomotor system, leading to changes in cortical regions that plan reading eye movements (including the frontal eye fields) [7]. The severity of the text-reading impairment is inversely proportional to the amount of visual field sparing to the right of fixation [2]. Fortunately, there have been several studies showing that eye-movement therapy can have a significant positive effect on text reading speed [8].

Read-Right was developed at UCL and funded by The Stroke Association. The aim was to provide patients with hemianopic alexia easy access to the therapy that had been shown to be effective in a previous, placebo-controlled, trial [1]. The site also includes testing materials: a visual field test that has been validated [9] and a standardized text reading test. An analysis of patients with right-sided hemianopias and hemianopic alexia using Read-Right, has shown that the web-based therapy worked at a group level, with similar effect sizes as seen in the original, phase II studies: ~40% average improvement after 15 hours of therapy and ~50% after 20 hours. This still leaves patients considerably away from their predicted pre-hemianopia reading speeds, but does seem to have an reasonable impact on their 'real world' reading ability with qualitative analysis showing that patients read an average of 30–60 min more per day [10].

Key Clinical Learning Points
- Homonymous hemianopias often persist, with little improvement after 6 months has passed
- Hemianopias affect many aspects of patients' lives, with reading impairment being common
- There is a good evidence base for eye-movement therapies in hemianopic alexia
- A free-to-use web-based therapy application is available to provide this therapy

References

1. Spitzyna GA, Wise RJ, McDonald SA, et al. Optokinetic therapy improves text reading in patients with hemianopic alexia: a controlled trial. Neurology. 2007;68(22):1922–30.
2. Zihl J. Eye movement patterns in hemianopic dyslexia. Brain. 1995;118:891–912.
3. Zhang X, Kedar S, Lynn MJ, et al. Natural history of homonymous hemianopia. Neurology. 2006;66(6):901–5.
4. Schofield TM, Leff AP. Rehabilitation of hemianopia. Curr Opin Neurol. 2009;22(1):36–40.
5. Schuett S, Heywood CA, Kentridge RW, et al. Rehabilitation of reading and visual exploration in visual field disorders: transfer or specificity? Brain. 2012;135(Pt 3):912–21.
6. Warren M. Pilot study on activities of daily living limitations in adults with hemianopsia. Am J Occup Ther. 2009;63(5):626–33.
7. Leff AP, Scott SK, Crewes H, et al. Impaired reading in patients with right hemianopia. Ann Neurol. 2000;47(2):171–8.
8. Schuett S. The rehabilitation of hemianopic dyslexia. Nat Rev Neurol. 2009;5(8):427–37.
9. Koiava N, Ong YH, Brown MM, et al. A 'web app' for diagnosing hemianopia. J Neurol Neurosurg Psychiatry. 2012;83(12):1222–4.
10. Ong YH, Brown MM, Robinson P, et al. Read-right: a "web app" that improves reading speeds in patients with hemianopia. J Neurol. 2012;259(12):2611–5.

Chapter 7
Recurrent Miscarriages and Neurological Symptoms

Deepa Arachchillage and Hannah Cohen

Clinical History

A 40-year-old female reported several episodes of transient visual loss, diplopia, loss of balance and worsening memory. She had also noted intermittent twitching of the facial muscles. There was no history of loss of consciousness or vomiting. She had a several year history of frequent migraine occurring two or three times weekly and helped by Migraleve™ (McNeil Healthcare, UK). In addition during her fourth pregnancy, aged 29, after three miscarriages in the second trimester, she developed chorea gravidarum and intermittent left sided facial numbness at 32 weeks gestation. During this pregnancy, she was treated with intermediate dose unfractionated heparin (UFH) (10,000 units bd with antenatal booking weight 70 kg) and high dose aspirin 150 mg daily started at 6 weeks gestation and continued throughout pregnancy. The pregnancy had a successful outcome with delivery at 38 weeks of gestation of a male infant of normal birth weight. The UFH was continued for 6 weeks postpartum and subsequently she was maintained on aspirin 75 mg daily.

There was no history of rheumatic fever in childhood and she was not on any regular medication prior to or after her successful pregnancy. An MRI brain scan post pregnancy was reported to show several areas of signal change, with uncertainty about the aetiology. The ANA was weakly positive and ds DNA negative. Investigations for antiphospholipid antibodies (aPL) showed a positive dilute Russell's viper venom time (DRVVT) test for lupus anticoagulant (LA), high

D. Arachchillage, MRCP, FRCPath
Haemostasis Research Unit, Department of Haematology,
University College London Hospitals NHS Foundation Trust and University
College London, London, UK

H. Cohen, MD, FRCP, FRCPath (✉)
Department of Haematology, University College London Hospitals
NHS Foundation Trust and University College London, London, UK
e-mail: hannah.cohen@uclh.nhs.uk

© Springer-Verlag London 2015
S.K. Gill et al. (eds.), *Stroke Medicine: Case Studies from Queen Square*,
DOI 10.1007/978-1-4471-6705-1_7

positive IgG anti beta 2 glycoprotein I (aβ2GPI) with IgG and IgM anticardiolipin antibodies (aCL) negative. Repeat investigations three months following this pregnancy showed persistently positive LA and high positive IgG anti beta 2 glycoprotein I (aβ2GPI). There was no history of joint symptoms, skin lesions or alopecia.

Aged 33, she developed episodes of transient visual loss, diplopia and loss of balance. An MRI brain scan at that stage was reported to show multiple small white matter lesions. She was therefore commenced on warfarin target INR 3.5 (range 3.0–4.0) and aspirin was stopped. She was on warfarin (target INR 3.5) with good anticoagulant management up to the time of the current symptoms.

Examination

She was alert and oriented. Fundoscopy and visual field examination were normal. Occasional twitching of the facial muscles was noted. There was no dysphasia. Tone and power were normal in all four limbs and both plantar responses were flexor. Although she had subjective sensory impairment over her left lower limb there was no objective evidence of sensory loss. A neuropsychological assessment indicated that she had impaired executive function, including lack of cognitive flexibility, difficulty with task switching and poor initiation and monitoring of actions. Examination of the cardiovascular and respiratory systems was normal.

Investigations

Repeat aPL testing confirmed a persistently positive LA with strongly positive IgG anti β2GPI. Both IgG and IgM aCL were negative as previously. Tests for autoantibodies including ANA, to extractable nuclear antigen (anti Ro anti La anti smooth muscle, anti Scl-70) and ds-DNA were negative.

An MRI brain scan revealed multiple white matter lesions in both frontal lobes in keeping with cerebral infarcts related to a small vessel arteriopathy (Fig. 7.1). Previous brain imaging was not available for comparison.

It was concluded that she had antiphospholipid syndrome (APS) with cerebral involvement.

Clinical Progress

In view of her new recent onset neurological symptoms, aspirin at a dose of 75 mg daily was added to the warfarin. A complication of a combination of warfarinisation and antiplatelet therapy was severe menorrhagia associated with iron deficiency

Fig. 7.1 Bilateral frontal lobes showing small white matter lesions in T2 weighted imaging. Multiple, presumed small cerebral infarcts are shown in the white matter of both frontal lobes

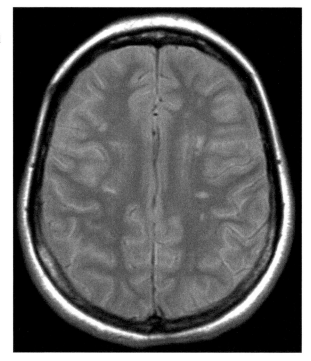

anaemia. At it's most severe she had a haemoglobin of 8.5 g/dL, which necessitates frequent INR monitoring to minimise the risk of over anticoagulation. Following insertion of a Mirena intrauterine device (IUD) her menorrhagia ceased. Due to continued neurological symptoms, despite warfarin plus aspirin, the aspirin was discontinued and dipyridamole (slow release) 200 mg twice daily substituted. Her neurological symptoms resolved completely on this regimen. She was managed in a multidisciplinary fashion during the course of her disease by haematologists, neurologists, obstetricians and gynaecologists.

Discussion

APS is characterised by thrombosis (arterial and/or venous and/or small vessel) and/or pregnancy morbidity, in association with persistently positive aPL. The updated international consensus (Sydney) classification laboratory criteria for definite APS require the presence of a LA and/or IgG or IgM aCL present in medium or high titre (i.e. >40 GPL or MPL or > the 99th percentile), and/or aβ2GPI (IgG and/or IgM) >99th percentile. These aPL should be persistent, defined as being present on two or more consecutive occasions at least 12 weeks apart [1]. These criteria were originally designed for scientific clinical studies and were not intended for diagnostic use.

Thrombotic APS is clinically heterogenous, manifesting with one or more episodes of thrombosis, which should be objectively diagnosed. APS-related pregnancy morbidity which may occur alone (obstetric APS) or in combination with thrombotic manifestations, defined in the Sydney criteria, includes recurrent miscarriages, unexplained death ≥10 weeks of a morphologically normal fetus or premature birth <34 weeks of a morphologically normal neonate because of severe pre-eclampsia/eclampsia or recognised features of placental insufficiency [1]. APS has been described as secondary if there is an associated autoimmune disorder, often systemic lupus erythematosus (SLE). However, the international consensus classification advises against using the term 'secondary' on the basis of that the relationship between APS and SLE is undefined [1].

Venous thromboembolism (VTE) in APS is most commonly manifests as lower limb deep vein thrombosis (DVT) and/or pulmonary embolism (PE). The most frequent site of arterial occlusion in APS, which may be thrombotic or embolic, is in the cerebral vasculature resulting in TIA or stroke. It has been observed that as many as 13% of ischaemic stroke and 7% of TIA are associated with aPL. However, aPL are common findings in the population and the association between aPL and stroke in the majority of stroke patients appears co-incidental. A large study has shown that the recurrence rate of stroke in unselected patients with stroke is identical in those with and without aPLs [2]. Thus, it is important to observe strict criteria for diagnosing APS and search for other causes of stroke even in individuals under 45 years. It has been estimated that the incidence of APS-related stroke is more than 20% [3]. However, this does not accord with our experience, which is that APS is a unusual cause of stroke, even in young patients.

The differential diagnosis includes other causes of a small vessel arteriopathy, including vasculitis, other autoimmune disorders (especially SLE) and hypertension.

Antithrombotic treatment is the mainstay treatment in patients with APS, but the optimal antithrombotic management for patients with APS-related stroke is uncertain because of lack of standardized laboratory tests to confirm the diagnosis of APS, limited data on its natural history, and a paucity of randomized treatment trials.

The revised international consensus (Sydney) classification criteria do not include other neurological manifestations which may be associated with aPL such as cognitive dysfunction, headache or migraine, multiple sclerosis-like disease, transverse myelitis, epilepsy, psychiatric disorders, ocular symptoms or chorea. Headache is one of the most often described neurologic manifestations in patients with APS presenting either a chronic headache or episodes of migraine, as experienced by our patient. There are incomplete and conflicting data on a possible relationship between migraine and aPL [4]. Cavestroc et al. reported in a comparative case study on 284 consecutive patients with migraine that those with migraine have a significantly higher prevalence of aPL, and suggested that the two conditions may be comorbid or even that migraine may be an early sign for identifying patients with aPL positivity [5]. Chorea gravidarum, i.e. chorea occurring during pregnancy or the early postpartum period, exhibited by our patient, is characterized by abrupt, brief, nonrhythmic, nonrepetitive movement of any limb, often associated with nonpatterned facial grimaces [3]. It is reported to be a rare neurologic manifestation in patients with APS. Chorea gravidarum may also be associated with oestrogen containing oral contraceptives [3]. This condition may be definable also as "pre APS" because it may antedate the appearance of thrombotic manifestations [3]. Sometimes symptoms presenting in APS patients can mimic multiple sclerosis (MS) especially symptoms related to balance and sensory symptoms. The MRI brain appearances of MS can mimic those of small vessel arteriopathies [3].

The British Committee for Standards in Haematology (BCSH) guidelines recommend that young adults (<50 years) with ischaemic stroke should be screened for aPL (2C) and for those with APS who may be at high risk of recurrence, warfarin should be considered [4]. The current mainstay of the treatment of venous and/or arterial thromboembolism in patients with APS is long term anticoagulation with warfarin or other vitamin K antagonists (VKA). For patients with a first episode of VTE or a recurrent VTE episode whilst off warfarin or at a sub-therapeutic INR, a target INR of 2.5 (range 2.0–3.0) is appropriate [4]. However, patients with arterial events and recurrent venous thrombosis whist on therapeutic anticoagulation were poorly represented in these studies, and therefore the optimal intensity of anticoagulation with VKA in these patient groups with APS is not established, although many experts in the field advise that they should be maintained at a target INR of >3.0 [6]. Anecdotal evidence suggests that some patients with non-criteria CNS manifestations, when associated with persistent aPL, may also benefit from anticoagulation [3]. Of note, our patient reported an improvement in migraine when she was anticoagulated for thrombotic APS. On the other hand, evidence for the benefit of anticoagulation is lacking. Thus, it might be appropriate to commence antiplatelet therapy initially and reserve anticoagulation for recurrent symptoms. Moreover, recurrent symptoms should always prompt review of the diagnosis and consideration of further investigations for other potential causes of small vessel vasculopathy.

There are limited therapeutic options for patients who have recurrent thrombotic events despite high intensity warfarin. These include addition of an antiplatelet agent, low molecular weight heparin (LMWH) including high intensity LMWH. The possibility that the INR may not reflect the true anticoagulant intensity should be considered. This is due to variable responsiveness of reagents used in the INR test to LA, leading to instability of anticoagulation [3, 7]. In this circumstance measurement of amidolytic factor X levels may be useful to assess the true intensity of anticoagulation of warfarin. There is a significantly higher risk of bleeding with high intensity anticoagulation with VKA [8] and with combined anticoagulant and antiplatelet treatment. The annual rate for bleeding events (fatal or non-fatal requiring hospital admission) with warfarin alone was 4.3% and for warfarin plus aspirin 5.1% [8]. Our patient experienced menorrhagia which necessitated frequent INR testing, to minimise periods of over anticoagulation and gynaecological input. Thrombosis is multifactorial and thus the presence of APS is likely to potentiate the risk of standard vascular risk factors for arterial thrombosis, such as hypertension and hyperlipidaemia which should be identified and actively managed. The risk of thrombosis is increased post-surgery and careful bridging anticoagulation is required.

In cases where anticoagulation has failed, empirical approaches include combining anticoagulation with immunosuppression and/or immunomodulation with modalities including rituximab, hydroxychloroquine, statins and complement inhibitors such as eculizumab [9]. The new oral anticoagulants (NOAC), dabigatran (a direct thrombin inhibitor), rivaroxaban, and apixaban (both factor Xa inhibitors) have shown promising results in the prevention of stroke and systemic embolism [7]. NOACs have also undergone phase III trials for the treatment of acute DVT and PE and secondary prevention of VTE and rivaroxaban has been licensed for these indications. NOAC represent a major therapeutic advance as, unlike warfarin, they do not require regular monitoring of their anticoagulant effects, do not interact with dietary constituents and alcohol and have few reported drug interactions [7]. There is currently an on-going prospective randomised controlled trial of warfarin versus rivartoxaban in patients with thrombotic APS with VTE (RAPS: Rivaroxaban in Antiphospholipid Syndrome) trial (http://isrctn.org/ISRCTN68222801). Subsequent appropriate studies are required to investigate the potential for use of these agents in stroke patients with APS.

Recurrent miscarriages, as occurred in this case are the most common obstetric complications in APS, although in the majority, these occur in the first trimester. Proven treatment for women with obstetric APS, in the absence of thrombosis, is antepartum administration of prophylactic or intermediate dose UFH or prophylactic LMWH combined with LDA, 75–100 mg/day [10].

This case illustrates the multisystem nature of APS and the requirement for careful attention to clinical and laboratory diagnosis and long term follow up. Optimal management necessitates a multidisciplinary approach, with input by various specialists including haematologists, neurologists, rheumatologists and obstetricians.

Key Clinical Learning Points

1. The diagnosis of APS requires persistently positive aPL, i.e. on two occasions at least 12 weeks apart in association with thrombosis (arterial and/or venous and/or small vessel) and/or pregnancy morbidity as defined in the updated (Sydney) international consensus classification criteria
2. The use and intensity of warfarin anticoagulation for arterial thrombosis in patients with APS is not evidence based. Many experts advise that high intensity warfarin ie. target INR 3.5 (range 3.0–4.0) should be used
3. Bleeding manifestations during treatment with high intensity anticoagulation should be actively managed
4. Proven treatment for women with obstetric APS is antepartum administration of prophylactic or intermediate dose UFH or prophylactic LMWH combined with low dose aspirin, 75–100 mg/day
5. Chorea and migraine are not included in the updated (Sydney) international consensus classification criteria for APS. Anecdotal reports suggest that a therapeutic trial of LMWH in selected patients with non-criteria manifestations prior to initiation of VKA, may be beneficial

Key Radiological Learning Points
1. It can be difficult to distinguish different underlying aetiology in patients with small vessel vasculopathy: white matter infarcts in APS, vasculitis and hypertensive small vessel disease can all look similar, as can inflammatory disorders, including MS

References

1. Miyakis S, Lockshin MD, Atsumi T, et al. International consensus statement on an update of the classification criteria for definite antiphospholipid syndrome (APS). J Thromb Haemost. 2006;4:295–306.
2. Panichpisal K, Rozner E, Levine SR. The management of stroke in antiphospholipid syndrome. Curr Rheumatol Rep. 2012;14:99–106.
3. Arnson Y, Shoenfeld Y, Alon E, et al. The antiphospholipid syndrome as a neurological disease. Semin Arthritis Rheum. 2010;40:97–108.
4. Keeling D, Mackie I, Moore GW, et al. British Committee for Standards in Haematology. Guidelines on the investigation and management of antiphospholipid syndrome. Br J Haematol. 2012;157:47–58.
5. Cavestro C, Micca G, Molinari F, et al. Migraineurs show a high prevalence of antiphospholipid antibodies. J Thromb Haemost. 2011;9:1350–4.
6. Ruiz-Irastorza G, Crowther M, Branch W, et al. Antiphospholipid syndrome. The Lancet. 2010;376:1498–509.
7. Arachchillage D, Cohen H. Use of new oral anticoagulants in antiphospholipid syndrome. Curr Rheumatol Rep. 2013;15(6):331.
8. Keeling D, Baglin T, Tait C, et al. British Committee for Standards in Haematology (BCSH) – guidelines for general haematology, haemostasis and thrombosis. Guidelines on oral anticoagulation with warfarin – fourth edition. Br J Haematol. 2011;154:311–24.
9. Erkan D, Rahman A, Cohen H, et al. What are the potential new treatments in antiphospholipid syndrome? In: Erkan D, Pierangeli S, editors. Antiphospholipid syndrome. London/New York: Springer; 2012.
10. Bates SM, Greer IA, Middeldorp S, et al. American College of Chest Physicians. VTE, thrombophilia, antithrombotic therapy, and pregnancy: Antithrombotic Therapy and Prevention of Thrombosis, 9th ed: American College of Chest Physicians Evidence-Based Clinical Practice Guidelines. Chest. 2012;141:e691S–736.

Chapter 8
A Pain in the Neck

Sumanjit K. Gill, Robert Simister, and David Collas

Clinical History

Whilst on the golf course, a 51-year old man developed sudden neck pain, dizziness, blurred vision, and unsteadiness. Two months of mild neck pain preceded these symptoms and he had been visiting an osteopath. He has no past medical history of note.

Examination

Upon arrival in the emergency department, his vital signs were normal with a BP of 120/80 mmHg. Systemic examination was normal. On neurological examination, he was drowsy, but was orientated in time and place. His pupils were equal and reactive to light and accommodation. There was nystagmus on leftward gaze. He was dysarthic. Cerebellar testing showed finger-nose ataxia on the left. Motor and sensory examination was normal, but he was unable to walk due to gait ataxia.

S.K. Gill, BSc Hons, MBBS, MRCP (✉)
Education Unit, National Hospital for Neurology and Neurosurgery,
UCL Institute of Neurology, London, UK
e-mail: sumanjit.gill@nhs.net

R. Simister, MA, FRCP, PhD
Comprehensive Stroke Service, National Hospital for Neurology and Neurosurgery,
UCLH Trust, London, UK

D. Collas, BSc, MBBS, FRCP
Stroke Medicine, Watford General Hospital, Watford, UK

© Springer-Verlag London 2015
S.K. Gill et al. (eds.), *Stroke Medicine: Case Studies from Queen Square*,
DOI 10.1007/978-1-4471-6705-1_8

Investigations and Clinical Progress

An initial CT scan was normal and thrombolysis was administered.

The neck pain subsided within one day. Ataxia, nausea and vertigo subsided over the next 24 hours, after which he was discharged home.

MRI and MR angiogram of the head and neck (Fig. 8.1) showed a left vertebral artery dissection. Mild tortuosity of the right vertebral artery was also noted.

Three days later he was on the golf course and had a recurrence of vertigo and ataxia on the left side. This resolved within 24 hours and he was started on a new oral anticoagulant drug due to concerns of residual clot within the dissection flap causing a transient ischaemic attack.

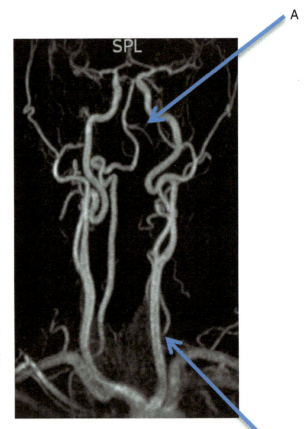

Fig. 8.1 Contrast enhanced MR angiogram showing (**a**) a short segment of the distal intradural left vertebral artery (presumed to fill retrogradely from the basilar artery) and (**b**) the attenuated proximal left vertebral artery with absent signal in the intervening vessel consistent with occlusion

Discussion

Vertebral dissection is a leading cause of stroke in young adults (age 18–45 years), and account for up to 25% of ischaemic stroke [1]. Spontaneous vertebral and carotid dissections cause approximately 2% of all strokes. Cerebral artery dissection was first described by Turnbull in 1915 but Fisher et al. were the first to clinically characterise spontaneous dissections in group of patients describing symptoms that varied from isolated headache to a complete hemiplegia [2]. Dissection can occur either apparently spontaneously or more commonly as a result of trauma. Detailed enquiry will often reveal a history of recent or simultaneous (sometimes trivial) cervical movement e.g. a sudden or excessive rotation or extension of the neck e.g. during yoga, painting the ceiling or as the result of a 'whiplash' injury in a car accident. This may have occurred some weeks prior to the infarct and often the history comes to light during the course of the admission or at follow up appointments. Amongst the conventional vascular risk factors, systemic hypertension is associated with an increased risk for neck artery dissection, whereas obesity, hyperlipidaemia and increasing age are associated with a decreased risk, perhaps because atherosclerosis protects against dissection. Cervical dissection is also associated with systemic conditions that disturb the integrity of blood vessel walls including fibromuscular dysplasia, Ehlers-Danlos, polyarteritis nodosa, Marfan syndrome, cystic medial necrosis, osteogenesis imperfecta, and polycystic kidney disease [3].

The vertebral artery (VA) is subdivided into four anatomical segments (Fig. 8.2). The proximal segment (V1) begins at the origin at the subclavian artery. Dissections typically occur at the junction between mobile and fixed segments ie at the V1-2 junction where the vertebral artery enters the transverse foramen, or more commonly, at the V2-3 segment, where the vessel emerges from its foramen to hooks over the transverse process of C2 and is particularly vulnerable to injury during neck rotation. The artery then penetrates the dura in the foramen magnum to become the fourth segment (V4) [4].

Pathologically [1], there are two possible underlying mechanisms for thrombosis. Firstly, a tear in the intima may lead to localised thrombosis in the lumen of the artery. In such cases, there may be no expansion of the wall by intramural bleeding and the diagnosis may rely only on the precipitation events associated with vertebral artery stenosis or occlusion on imaging. Secondly, there may be bleeding into the wall of artery (i.e. true dissection of the artery), either via an intimal tear or as a result of traumatic or spontaneous bleeding from adventitial vessels in the wall of the artery. The haematoma in the wall can then be seen on cross-sectional imaging of the artery and may compress the lumen resulting in slow flow, thrombosis or occlusion of the vessel. TIA or ischaemic stroke can then occur either as a result of propagation of thrombus to distal branches or as a result of 'artery to artery embolism' or as a result of impaired flow, especially if the involved VA is 'dominant' ie associated with a very small or absent contralateral VA.

Clinical features of VA dissection are sometimes subtle and asymptomatic dissection is occasionally found as an incidental finding on vascular imaging done

Fig. 8.2 CT Angiogram (normal appearances) annotated to demonstrate segments of the vertebral arteries and their terminal branches [6]

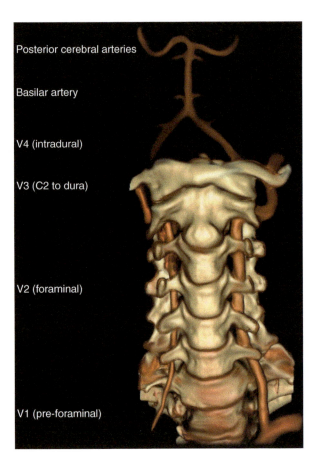

Posterior cerebral arteries

Basilar artery

V4 (intradural)

V3 (C2 to dura)

V2 (foraminal)

V1 (pre-foraminal)

for an unrelated reason. Unilateral posterior neck pain and occipital headache can be a prominent feature and may occur in isolation. In such cases, the symptoms might easily be dismissed as musculoskeletal or as migraine, especially in younger patients in the absence of conventional risk factors. The symptoms of ischaemia or infarction secondary to vertebral artery dissection are very varied because emboli can migrate to arteries supplying the cerebellum, brain stem, thalamus or in the distribution of one or both posterior cerebral arteries. Patients may also present with subarachnoid or parenchymal haemorrhage if the dissection extends intradurally because the intradural V4 segment is thin-walled and can easily rupture [2].

The diagnosis of vertebral artery dissection on vascular imaging is not always straightforward. A constriction of the VA may reflect arterial dissection, but can

Fig. 8.3 Axial T2 weighted fat saturated image showing high signal crescent-shaped mural haematoma in the wall of the left vertebral (*arrow*) pathognomic of arterial dissection. Fat saturation annuls surrounding high signal from fat in the neck to improve conspicuity of the haematoma

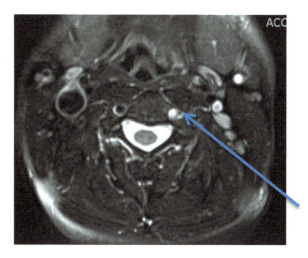

also reflect atherosclerosis, radiation therapy or a congenitally small VA. Cross-sectional cervical MRI with fat-suppressed images have become important in demonstrating haematoma in the arterial wall pathognomic of dissection [1]. However, there are often challenges differentiating blood from perivascular fat or venous plexus. CTA can be more specific in demonstrating true expansion of the artery with crescentic mural high density or an apparent 'double lumen'. Imaging may show pseudo-aneurysm formation, particularly where dissection involves the V4 segment. Catheter angiography may still be indicated to detect/confirm subtle dissections or discriminate dissection from other causes of stenosis. Re-imaging at around 3 months after onset may be helpful in confirming the diagnosis if remodelling of the artery and/or absorption of an intramural haematoma can be demonstrated. Serial imaging is also required where pseudoaneurysm is present, to monitor for expansion because of the risk of rupture (Fig. 8.3).

Patients with VA dissection are routinely treated with antiplatelet therapy or anticoagulation with the aim of preventing recurrent stroke. Observational studies suggest that there is no difference in the effectiveness of antiplatelet and anticoagulant therapy in preventing recurrent stroke or death, with relatively low rates of recurrence once the diagnosis is established and patients are started on treatment. Choice of agent may be influenced by factors such as the extent of cerebral infarction and intradural dissection into the V4 segment, with risk of subarachnoid haemorrhage, often considered a contraindication to anticoagulation [5].

The overall clinical outcome is usually good with a low risk of lasting disability, especially in young patients. The risk of recurrent stroke is highest in the first month at around 2% with an annual risk of around 1% thereafter. Other factors influencing outcome include the calibre of the contralateral vertebral artery and integrity of the circle of Willis.

Key Clinical Learning Points
1. Vertebral artery dissection is a leading cause of posterior circulation stroke in younger patients
2. Unilateral neck pain and/or occipital headache are often features in the presenting symptoms
3. Anticoagulation can be given in the acute phase if the risk of bleeding is low enough for it to be safely administered: consider the systemic bleeding risk, the size of the associated infarct and whether there is any risk of intradural extension

Key Radiological Learning Points
1. The diagnosis of VA dissection can be challenging and may require a combination of MRI/A, CTA and occasionally catheter angiography
2. The intramural haematoma is often seen on CT/MR imaging as a 'double lumen' or a crescent shape in the vessel wall associated with expansion of the artery
3. The typical site of dissection is in the V2 and V3 segments of the VA at the junction between fixed and mobile arterial segments

References

1. Scheivink WI. Spontaneous dissection of the carotid and vertebral arteries. N Engl J Med. 2001;344(12):898–906.
2. Fisher CM, Ojemann RG, Roberson GH. Spontaneous dissection of cervico-cerebral arteries. Can J Neurol Sci. 1978;5(1):9–19.
3. Debette S, Leys D. Cervical-artery dissections: predisposing factors, diagnosis, and outcome. Lancet Neurol. 2009;8:668–78.
4. Cloud GC, Markus HS. Diagnosis and management of vertebral stenosis. Q J Med. 2003;96:27–34.
5. Kennedy F, Lanfranconi S, Hicks C, et al. Antiplatelets versus anticoagulation for dissection. Neurology. 2013;80:970–1.
6. http://en.wikipedia.org/wiki/Vertebral_artery. Accessed on 13/01/2014.

Chapter 9
A Painless Loss of Vision

David Doig and Fiona Kennedy

Clinical History

A 49-year-old right-handed lady attended a 'Rapid Access TIA' clinic at a Hyperacute Stroke Unit (HASU). The previous morning, the patient had awoken with painless loss of vision in her right eye. She was systemically well and did not have any other symptoms. She was not on any medication but was a current smoker. She did not have any other vascular risk factors.

Examination

On examination the right pupil was not reactive to light and there was no perception of light, except for a thin temporal crescent. Examination of the left eye was normal including visual field examination. Extra-ocular movements were normal and the remaining cranial nerves intact. Power, tone, co-ordination, sensation and reflexes were normal in the upper and lower limbs. Cardiovascular examination revealed normal heart sounds and a regular pulse of 70 bpm. Blood pressure on admission was 170/86 mmHg. A 12 lead ECG showed normal sinus rhythm. At this point in the assessment the patient was loaded with 300 mg Aspirin and then commenced on Clopidogrel 75 mg. She was diagnosed as having right central retinal artery occlusion and admitted to the HASU for further investigation.

D. Doig, MBChB, BScMedSci (Hons), MRCP (✉)
F. Kennedy, MB, Bch, BAO, MRCP (UK)
Stroke Research Group, Department of Brain Repair and Rehabilitation, UCL Institute of Neurology, University College London, National Hospital for Neurology and Neurosurgery, London, UK
e-mail: d.doig@ucl.ac.uk; fiona.kennedy@ucl.ac.uk

© Springer-Verlag London 2015
S.K. Gill et al. (eds.), *Stroke Medicine: Case Studies from Queen Square*,
DOI 10.1007/978-1-4471-6705-1_9

Investigations

CT scan of the brain did not show any abnormality but CTA revealed a tight stenosis of the right ICA. On the CTA there was a long segment-filling defect of the proximal cervical ICA from its origin. She went onto have a carotid ultrasound to confirm the stenosis in the right ICA. This showed a patient right ICA with heterogeneous plaque, including some soft material, at the origin causing an 80–89% stenosis (Fig. 9.1). However, distal to the origin there was the appearance of flow through soft material in the lumen, consistent with the presence of thrombus in the artery. There was no significant stenosis noted in the left ICA and both vertebral arteries were normal.

With the results of the carotid ultrasound in hand, the patient was anti-coagulated with dalteparin. The vascular team assessed the patient but there was a high risk of causing a stroke if they operated on a patient with ICA stenosis and fresh clot in the vessel. The plan is made to continue with anti-coagulation and repeat the ultrasound after 2–3 days treatment.

There was no obvious thrombus on the repeat ultrasound however there was still evidence of heterogeneous plaque in the ICA causing an 80–89% stenosis.

MRI/MRA was performed and was reported as showing an established area of cortical damage overlying the right inferior parietal lobule in the region of the right MCA/PCA borderzone which was thought to represent a small cortical borderzone infarct. The MRA showed a 90% stenosis of the right carotid bifurcation (Fig. 9.2).

The patient continued on anti-coagulation and was discharged from the hospital with regular follow up and repeat ultrasound in the vascular clinic.

After 8 weeks the patient was randomised in a carotid artery trial, the 2nd European Carotid Surgery Trial (ECST-2). In this trial patients with asymptomatic or symptomatic carotid artery disease who have a low to intermediate risk of recurrent stroke are randomised between 'immediate revascularisation and optimal medial therapy' or 'optimal medical therapy alone'. The patient consented to the trial and was randomised to 'immediate revascularisation' and had a carotid endarterectomy 8 weeks after her presenting retinal stroke. Unfortunately one month follow up MRI and carotid ultrasound showed that she had occluded her right ICA post-CEA, but this was asymptomatic.

Discussion

The finding of free-floating thrombus (FFT) in the common or internal carotid artery (ICA) is uncommon, but the condition has been well-described since the introduction of arterial imaging that makes the diagnosis possible.

Patients most commonly present symptomatically with a fragment of thrombus breaking off, embolising distally, and causing cerebral or ocular ischaemia or infarction. This patient suffered a right central artery occlusion causing unilateral loss of

Fig. 9.1 Carotid Doppler
ultrasound showing soft
intraluminal thrombus
extending cranially from an
underlying atherosclerotic
plaque in the right carotid
artery

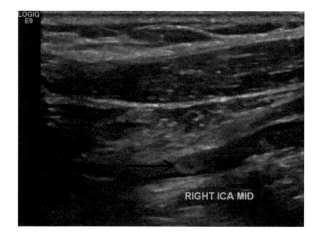

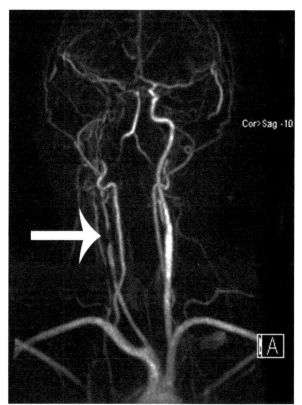

Fig. 9.2 Contrast-enhanced
magnetic resonance
angiogram showing severe
stenosis of the right ICA
(*arrowed*)

vision. There is often a temporal crescent of preserved vision in central retinal occlusion as here the retina is very thin and can be perfused from the choroidal circulation. The detection of asymptomatic carotid thrombus is rare, being discovered as part of screening for vascular disease elsewhere, following the discovery of a carotid bruit on clinical examination, or as part of pre-operative workup for procedures such as cardiac bypass grafting and valve replacement surgery [1].

In patients with cerebral or ocular symptoms attributable to embolic disease the incidence of FFT on carotid imaging is estimated to be <1% across non-invasive imaging techniques. The diagnosis is more common in men than women, and the most common underlying aetiology is ulcerated or ruptured carotid atheroma [2]. Other possible causes include carotid dissection, hypercoagulable state or a thrombus from the left side of the heart lodging in the ICA. Additionally, the condition has been described in association with cancer chemotherapeutic agents, which may cause endothelial injury and platelet activation [3].

The diagnosis of FFT is made on vascular imaging. Definitions vary, but one proposed set of criteria are the appearance of "elongated thrombus attached to the arterial wall with circumferential blood flow at its distal most aspect with cyclical motion relating to cardiac cycles" [2].

Arterigography

Non-invasive investigation with CT or MR contrast angiography is preferred over intra-arterial catheter angiogram because of the potential for causing stroke during the latter procedure. Although that risk is low, high resolution CT or MR may be able to demonstrate the typical appearance of FFT with lower morbidity. A characteristic "doughnut sign" is described where an intraluminal filling defect is surrounded by a ring of enhancement inside the vessel [4]. On sagittal or coronal reformatted images this may appear as a filling defect extending towards the distal end of the vessel. MR with additional sequences may also be able to demonstrate a dissection. However, although these modalities are able to demonstrate the full length of the carotid from aortic origin to the circle of Willis, they are not able to demonstrate whether the filling defect is mobile, and additional imaging may be required in the form of ultrasound.

Ultrasound

Carotid Doppler ultrasound (DUS) is a low-cost and well-tolerated alternative to CTA or MRA. Ultrasound may be able to identify an underlying atherosclerotic plaque or arterial dissection, and crucially can visualize the thrombus over time showing cyclical motion of a clot. Since ultrasound relies on blood flow velocity for the diagnosis of carotid stenosis, the presence of soft thrombus which may absorb some of the kinetic energy of the circulation may cause underestimation of the severity of underlying atherosclerosis [5]. It may therefore be necessary to repeat DUS after resolution of the thrombus.

Management Options

A conservative approach to management employs ether antiplatelet or anticoagulant drugs to prevent propagation of the thrombus and promote its resolution by the normal fibrinolytic pathways in the blood. Serial angiographic studies of patients with FFT have shown resolution of the thrombus on medical therapy alone [6]. The best available guidance for which treatment to use comes from the carotid dissection literature. Currently, only small-scale studies comparing antiplatelet with anticoagulant therapy have been reported, and meta-analysis of these studies has failed to show a difference in the rate of stroke or death on either treatment [7].

CEA is an attractive alternative to medical therapy; after distal clamping of the carotid is achieved during CEA the clot can be removed in its entirety without fear of distal embolization. Good surgical results have been reported in case series [8]. However, concern remains that handling of the artery prior to clamping may dislodge clot.

A number of interventional neuroradiological approaches to the management of FFT have been described. These include the deployment of a stent to "trap" the thrombus in the stent [3, 9], aspiration by suction thrombectomy [3] and "stabilization" of the thrombus by coil embolization of the ICA [3]. It is possible that this approach carries a higher risk than surgery as during most interventional procedures flow in the carotid is maintained, so any particulate debris dislodged by manipulation of the guidewire or catheter may embolise to the brain. Strategies to decrease the risk of this occurring include the placement of a cerebral protection device, balloon occlusion of the artery to produce flow arrest, or using a flow-reversal device. The long-term outcomes of these approaches remain unknown.

Key Clinical Learning Points
- Free-floating thrombus (FFT) in the carotid artery is rare but important to diagnose as there are treatment options available
- There is no clear evidence-based consensus on the management of free-floating thrombus in the carotid artery
- Medical therapy consists of antiplatelet or anticoagulant drugs
- Surgical management consists of either carotid endarterectomy or a percutaneous interventional procedure

Key Radiological Learning Points
- Imaging appearances on non-invasive angiography may include the so-called "doughnut sign" or other intraluminal filling defect surrounded by intravenous contrast
- Ultrasound can demonstrate mobile thrombus and may help identify an underlying pathology such as dissection or atherosclerotic plaque
- Serial non-invasive imaging may confirm resolution of the thrombus and reveal an underlying stenosis or dissection

References

1. Csobay-Novák C, Járányi Z, Dósa E, et al. Asymptomatic free-floating thrombus of the internal carotid artery. Interv Med Appl Sci. 2011;3(4):213–5.
2. Bhatti A, Leon Jr LR, Labropoulos N, et al. Free-floating thrombus of the carotid artery: literature review and case reports. J Vasc Surg. 2007;45:199–205.
3. Park JW, Lee DH, Choi CG, et al. Various endovascular approaches to the management of free floating carotid thrombi: a technical report. J Neurointerv Surg. 2012;4:336–8.
4. Jaberi A, Lum C, Stefanski P, et al. Computed tomography angiography evaluation of internal carotid artery free-floating thrombus: single-center diagnosis, false-positives, and follow-up. Emerg Radiol. 2012;19:359–62.
5. Chua HC, Lim T, Teo BC, et al. Free-floating thrombus of the carotid artery detected on carotid ultrasound in patient with cerebral infarcts: a 10-year study. Ann Acad Med. 2012;41(9):420–4.
6. Pelz DM, Buchan A, Fox AJ, et al. Intraluminal thrombus of the internal carotid arteries: angiographic demonstration of resolution with anticoagulant therapy alone. Radiology. 1986;160:369–73.
7. Kennedy F, Lanfranconi C, Hicks C, et al. Antiplatelets vs anticoagulation for dissection. CADISS nonrandomized arm and meta-analysis. Neurology. 2012;79(7):686–9.
8. Lane TRA, Shalhoub J, Perera R, et al. Diagnosis and surgical management of free-floating thrombus within the carotid artery. Vasc Endovascular Surg. 2010;44:586–93.
9. Tummala RP, Jahromi BS, Yamamoto J, et al. Carotid artery stenting under flow arrest for the management of intraluminal thrombus: technical case report. Oper Neurosurg. 2008;63(ONS Suppl 1):ONSE89–90.

Chapter 10
Sickle Cell Disease and Stroke

Georgios Niotakis and Vijeya Ganesan

Clinical History

A 3-year-old Nigerian girl, with previously uncomplicated sickle cell disease (HbSS) developed an unprovoked acute left hemiparesis and aphasia. She was treated with an urgent exchange transfusion and thereafter continued on a regular transfusion programme. However, despite blood transfusions every 3–4 weeks her HbS level was never less than 40%; transfusion therapy was limited by difficulties with vascular access. Unfortunately, she developed further neurological symptoms, with recurrent episodes of dysphasia and an episode of acute right hemiparesis, one year after the first event. Aspirin and hydroxyurea were prescribed.

Examination

Neurological examination showed minimal long tract signs on the right and normal cognitive function.

Investigations

She was referred for a sleep study that showed episodes of nocturnal desaturation and, following ear, nose and throat consultation, she underwent adenotonsillectomy.

G. Niotakis
Paediatric Neurology, Great Ormond Street Hospital for Children, London, UK

V. Ganesan, MRCPCH, MD (✉)
Neurosciences Unit, UCL Institute of Child Health, London, UK
e-mail: v.ganesan@ucl.ac.uk

© Springer-Verlag London 2015   63
S.K. Gill et al. (eds.), *Stroke Medicine: Case Studies from Queen Square*,
DOI 10.1007/978-1-4471-6705-1_10

Brain MRI and MRA was repeated at this time; there were bilateral borderzone infarcts (Fig. 10.1) and a severe occlusive arteriopathy affecting both terminal internal carotid arteries, with basal "moyamoya" collaterals (Fig. 10.2).

She was referred for consideration of revascularisation surgery. It was felt that this should be deferred until her medical management could be optimised, hence an indwelling central venous line ("portacath") was inserted, which facilitated effective blood transfusion. With HbS levels consistently <30% and Hb >10 g/dl she has remained clinically and radiologically stable.

Discussion

Arterial ischaemic stroke (AIS) affects at least 10% of children with sickle cell disease (SCD) by 20 years of age and has a >60% recurrence rate without intervention [1]. Up to 25% of people with HbSS phenotype have ischaemic brain injury on MRI – so called "silent infarcts" that, nonetheless, have adverse effects on cognition. Many risk factors are implicated in AIS associated with SCD, including cerebral arteriopathy, anaemia, chronic hypoxaemia, prior chest crisis and high white cell count. Obstructive airways disease (from big tonsils and adenoids), infections, patent foramen ovale and relative hypertension are modifiable risk factors associated with AIS in children with SCD – immunization and penicillin prophylaxis has decreased the prevalence of bacterial meningitis with subsequent stroke.

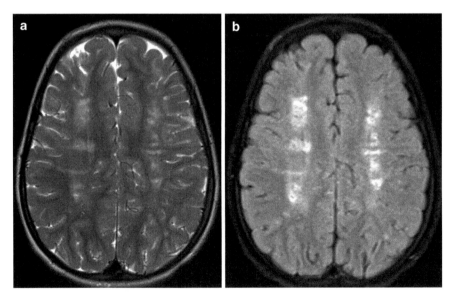

Fig. 10.1 Axial (**a**) T2-weighted and (**b**) FLAIR images from the patient described above showing bilateral deep borderzone infarcts, typical of the distribution of cerebral infarction in SCD

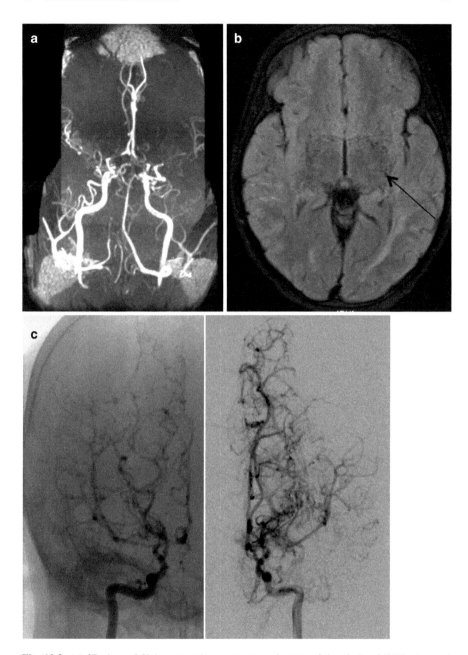

Fig. 10.2 (**a**) 2D time-of-flight magnetic resonance angiogram of the circle of Willis (coronal projection), showing an occlusive arteriopathy affecting both terminal ICAs and proximal MCAs and ACAs. The typical "moyamoya" collaterals are better appreciated on (**b**) the axial T1-weighted image, as flow voids in the basal ganglia (*arrow*) and on (**c**) the cerebral angiogram (*right & left* ICA injections, frontal projection)

The intracranial occlusive cerebral arteriopathy in SCD primarily affects the terminal ICA, proximal MCA and ACAs – i.e. large intracranial arteries [1]. The genesis of the arteriopathy is complex and factors such as the interaction between the abnormal red cells and the arterial endothelium are implicated. Large vessel arteriopathy is present in the vast majority of patients who develop AIS. Some develop a "moyamoya" morphology (with basal collaterals identical to those seen in idiopathic moyamoya disease), which predicts a high rate of AIS recurrence despite conventional SCD AIS prophylactic strategies.

The STOP trial showed that screening children with SCD for arteriopathy using TCD to measure flow velocity in the MCA, and then offering prophylactic blood transfusion to those with elevated MCA velocity was highly effective in primary prevention of AIS in SCD [2]. MCA velocity >200 cm/s is the strongest known risk factor for stroke in SCD [3]. The NHS Sickle Cell and Thalassaemia Screening Programme [4] and the American Heart Association [1] recommend that all children with SCD are offered TCD screening annually between the ages of 2 and 16 years.

TCD results are considered normal if MCA velocity is <170 cm/s, "conditional" (170–200 cm/s), or abnormal if >200 cm/s [4]. Transfusion if recommended for those with MCA velocity >200 cm/s; those with conditional TCD results should have a repeat TCD between 1 and 4 months later, especially in young children. It is important to be aware that MCA velocity <70 cm/s might indicate severe occlusive disease, and these patients should be investigated with CTA or MRA. Recently it has emerged that a high proportion of SCD patients with AIS have cervical arteriopathy – the aetiology of this remains unclear but includes arterial dissection in some cases.

Exchange transfusion is recommended for management of acute AIS in SCD [1]. AIS is an indication for on-going periodic transfusions, with the aim of maintaining HbS levels < 30% and suppressing erythropoiesis by maintaining Hb >10 g/dl [1, 4]. Blood transfusion is a highly onerous intervention, with the risk of blood borne infection, antibody formation, vascular access and iron overload. Chelation therapy is important in the prevention of iron overload, and this can now be achieved using oral agents. The STOP2 trial established that the protective effects of transfusion are only maintained while transfusion is continued, hence the duration of transfusion therapy remains relatively open ended.

Hydroxyurea (or Hydroxycarbamide) increases HbF, which protects against AIS. Although hydroxyurea was not superior to transfusion in a clinical trial [3], the inaccessibility of transfusion to many children with SCD to makes this a potential option for AIS prevention in resource poor settings. Aspirin is widely used in childhood AIS prevention and may have a role in SCD arteriopathy; however the risk of haemorrhagic stroke is increased in children with SCD and aspirin may further increase this risk [1].

Only haematopoietic stem cell transplantation offers potentially curative treatment for SCD, ideally from a HLA-matched family donor [5]. There are major risks including infection, graft versus host disease, failure to engraft, growth failure and death. In the UK and USA AIS is an indication for stem cell transplantation in SCD.

There have been several series describing successful revascularisation surgery in children with moyamoya and SCD [6]. The AHA recommends revascularisation "as a last resort" [1] and the role of this intervention in the context of conventional AIS prophylaxis in SCD is not established. Our own practice is to consider revascularisation in children who have a moyamoya-like arteriopathy and who continue to be clinically or radiologically symptomatic despite blood transfusion. We consider surgery an adjunctive strategy and advocate continuing with conventional management, including transfusion.

Key Clinical Learning Points
1. AIS is common in children with SCD, with a high rate of recurrence
2. Blood transfusion is highly effective in preventing AIS recurrence
3. AIS is an indication for bone marrow transplantation in SCD
4. Other potential adjunctive treatments include hydroxyurea, treatment of hypertension, nocturnal hypoxaemia, aspirin and surgical revascularisation

---

Key Radiological Learning Points
1. Cerebral infarction typically affects the deep borderzone regions in the white matter, especially in the frontal regions in SCD (Fig. 10.1)
2. Most AIS in SCD is secondary to occlusive intracranial large vessel arteriopathy
3. Moyamoya-like arteriopathy is predictive of an aggressive clinical course, with a high rate of recurrence (Fig. 10.2)
4. Cervical arteriopathy is increasingly identified in SCD
5. AIS is preventable by blood transfusion in those with abnormal TCD results; TCD screening should be undertaken in all children aged >2 years

References

1. Roach ES, Golomb MR, Adams R, et al. Management of stroke in infants and children: a scientific statement from a special writing group of American Heart Association Stroke Council and the Council on Cardiovascular Disease in the Young. Stroke. 2008;39:2644–91.
2. Jordan LC, Casella JF, DeBaun MR. Prospects for primary stroke prevention in children with sickle cell anaemia. Br J Haematol. 2012;157:14–25.
3. Ware RE, Schultz WH, Yovetich N, et al. Stroke with Transfusions Changing to Hydroxyurea (SWiTCH): a phase III randomised controlled trial for treatment of children with sickle cell anemia, stroke, and iron overload. Pediatr Blood Cancer. 2011;57:1011–7.
4. Dick M for the UK Forum on Haemoglobin Disorders. Sickle cell disease in childhood: standards and guidelines for clinical care. NHS Sickle Cell and Thalassaemia Screening Programme in partnership with the Sickle Cell Society. London. October 2012.
5. Hsieh MM, Fitzhugh CD, Tisdale JF, et al. Allogeneic heamtopoietic stem cell transplantation for sickle cell disease: the time is now. Blood. 2011;118:1197–207.
6. Smith ER, McClain CD, Heeney M, et al. Pial synangiosis in patients with moyamoya syndrome and sickle cell anemia: perioperative management and surgical outcome. Neurosurg Focus. 2009;26(4):E10.

Chapter 11
A New Mother with Rapidly Developing Blindness

David Collas

Clinical History

A 17-year-old woman first presented to the Accident and Emergency department 5 days after the birth of her first child complaining of a severe headache. This had begun gradually and became throbbing in nature, and was predominantly left sided. There was no history of migraine, nausea, vomiting, fever or neck stiffness. Her recent birth had been an uncomplicated vaginal delivery of her first child. She was known to be heterozygous for Factor V Leiden and her mother had a history of thrombophilia. On examination the Accident and Emergency department on this first visit, she has an elevated blood pressure of 180/100 but no other abnormalities. Laboratory investigations were also normal; in particular there was no proteinuria. She was discharged with a diagnosis of migraine.

Two days later she returned the Accident and Emergency department with steadily deteriorating visual acuity, which had progressed over the preceding 12 hours to the extent that she could only perceive hand movements. In the Accident and Emergency department she had a generalised tonic-clonic seizure, which was terminated with magnesium and diazepam. She was also given a loading dose of phenytoin.

Examination

On examination she was drowsy. Her visual acuity was reduced to perception of hand movements, but her pupillary responses and fundi were normal. She had bilateral extensor plantar responses and brisk reflexes, which were particularly marked

D. Collas, BSc, MB, BS FRCP
Stroke Medicine, Watford General Hospital, Watford, UK
e-mail: david.collas@whht.nhs.uk

© Springer-Verlag London 2015
S.K. Gill et al. (eds.), *Stroke Medicine: Case Studies from Queen Square*,
DOI 10.1007/978-1-4471-6705-1_11

in the left arm. Tone, power and coordination were normal. Her BP remained elevated at 180/100. The differential diagnoses considered were intracerebral haemorrhage, cerebral infarction, cerebral venous sinus thrombosis, eclampsia and posterior reversible encephalopathy syndrome.

Investigations

CT brain (Fig. 11.1) showed effacement of the sulci bilaterally at the posterior poles and low attenuation in the right occipital lobe, suggestive of early bilateral infarction. There was no evidence of haemorrhage. MRI showed extensive areas of high signal on FLAIR bilaterally (Fig. 11.2) with minimal signal change on DWI (B1000 right occipital lobe, Fig. 11.3), indicative of vasogenic rather than cytotoxic oedema. This was confirmed on the ADC map which shows increased, rather than reduced diffusion, excluding cerebral infarction. MR venogram excluded venous sinus thrombosis.

Clinical Progress

A diagnosis was made of posterior reversible encephalopathy syndrome (PRES) secondary to post-partum eclampsia. She received treatment with intravenous labetolol to lower blood pressure as a priority, attaining a stable level of 140/80, and was continued on oral phenytoin. Her response to treatment was dramatic, with vision returning to near normal acuity within a few days, and a persistent area of blurred vision in the left hemi-field resolved a few days later. Her headaches improved and by 8 weeks after onset she had recovered completely. A follow up MRI was normal and all the acute abnormalities had disappeared.

Discussion

The postpartum period is accompanied by an increased risk of both ischaemic and haemorrhagic stroke from various mechanisms, including hypertension of pregnancy, eclampsia, cerebral venous thrombosis and post-partum vasculitis. The syndrome of PRES was described in 1996 [1], and comprises blindness, seizures, altered consciousness, and headache occurring in the context of raised blood pressure. As the name implies, the term PRES refers primarily to the radiological appearance of reversible oedema in the posterior circulation associated with impaired consciousness or confusion. The majority of cases show at least some of the clinical features of hypertensive encephalopathy [2] or if the patient is pregnant

Fig. 11.1 CT (2 window levels) demonstrates focal low density and swelling of right occipital pole brain tissue

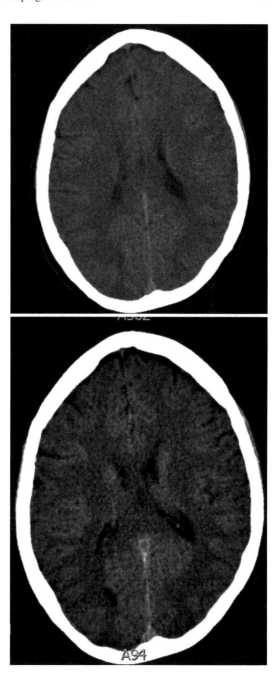

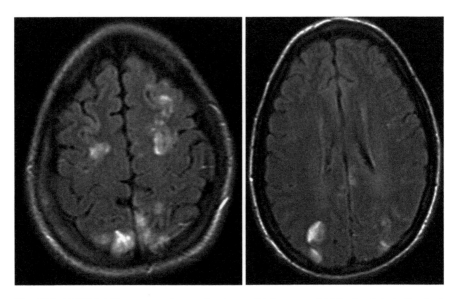

Fig. 11.2 MRI FLAIR sequence image showing multiple areas of high signal including both parieto-occipital regions and both frontal lobes i.e. in anterior and posterior cerebral circulation territories

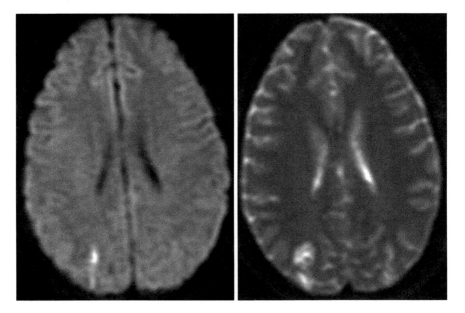

Fig. 11.3 DWI B1000 and ADC map imaging demonstrating high signal in corresponding parietal areas on both studies suggesting vasogenic rather than cytotoxic oedema and excluding acute infarction

or in the post-partum period, eclampsia as this case illustrates. However, the full-blown picture of hypertensive encephalopathy or eclampsia may not be present (e.g. as in this case, there may be no papilloedema and no renal involvement). Other provoking circumstances include renal dialysis and chemotherapy. Similar clinical and radiological features can also be seen in the reversible vasoconstriction syndrome (see case 34). Thus the term PRES should always be accompanied by a diagnosis of the precipitating condition and investigations should include angiographic imaging and venography.

The mechanism of the reversible changes in PRES appears to be increased vascular permeability, which is usually confined to, or most severe in the posterior circulation, caused by endothelial injury and impaired autoregulation [3]. The vasogenic oedema results in the encephalopathy associated with acute deterioration of vision from involvement of the visual cortex in the occipital lobes. However, as illustrated in this case, the radiological appearances of PRES and the clinical features of more widespread cortical involvement are not necessarily confined to the posterior circulation. Untreated, the persistence of uncontrolled hypertension and continuing seizures will result in permanent neuronal damage, probably through impairment of the microcirculation or secondary thrombosis secondary to endothelial injury. If infarction occurs in the context of PRES, cytotoxic oedema will occur and complicate the radiological picture. Strictly speaking, PRES is no longer reversible (and therefore not an appropriate description) if infarction occurs, which illustrates that the importance of restricting the term to a radiological description, as well as the importance of early management.

Key Clinical Learning Points
1. There is an increased risk of ischaemic and haemorrhagic stroke related to pregnancy, which persists for 4–6 weeks after delivery
2. PRES is a radiological diagnosis and should be accompanied by a diagnosis of the precipitating condition
3. Postpartum seizures and raised blood pressure are a feature of eclampsia, which may cause PRES in the absence of proteinuria or papilloedema
4. Prompt control of blood pressure is crucial to reduce the risk of permanent damage in both eclampsia and other causes of PRES [4]. Labetolol is preferred to vasodilators as these might exacerbate the pathophysiology changes underlying PRES
5. Despite the dramatic presentation with fits and blindness, prompt intervention as described can achieve full recovery. The most important factor is that the condition is recognised early and effectively treated

Key Radiological Learning Points

1. CT imaging should be performed to detect haemorrhage or infarction and should include contrast angiography, both venous and arterial

2. The finding of extensive high signal on FLAIR not confined to any one vascular area is suggestive of non-arterial pathology [5]. Low signal on DWI or T2 shine-through (as indicated by increased signal on ADC map instead of low signal) indicates vasogenic oedema. This differentiates it from the cytotoxic oedema of early infarction, and carries a different differential diagnosis, including PRES

3. The context of the presentation, such as pregnancy, postpartum period, dialysis or chemotherapy is an important pointer to the correct interpretation of the scans leading to the correct diagnosis

4. Vasogenic oedema also occurs in a wide variety of other conditions apart from PRES, of which the commonest is tumour

References

1. Hinchey J, Chaves C, Appignani B, et al. A reversible posterior leuko-encephalopathy syndrome. N Engl J Med. 1996;334:494–500.
2. Schwartz RB. Hyperperfusion encephalopathies: hypertensive encephalopathy and related conditions. Neurologist. 2002;8:22–34.
3. Haubrich C, Wendt A, Diehl RR, et al. Dynamic autoregulation testing in the posterior cerebral artery. Stroke. 2004;35:848–52.
4. Striano P, Striano S, Tortora F, et al. Clinical spectrum and critical care management of Posterior Reversible Encephalopathy Syndrome (PRES). Med Sci Monit. 2005;11: CR549–53.
5. Casey SO, Sampaio RC, Michel E, et al. Posterior reversible encephalopathy syndrome: utility of fluid-attenuated inversion recovery MR imaging in the detection of cortical and subcortical lesions. AJNR Am J Neuroradiol. 2000;21:1199–206.

Chapter 12
A Potentially Fatal Complication

Victoria Wykes, Daniel Epstein, and Joan P. Grieve

Clinical History

A 49-year-old right-handed male bus driver presented to the emergency department with sudden onset of left sided weakness commencing at 1 pm whilst eating lunch. His colleague noticed these symptoms, promptly called an ambulance and he arrived in the emergency department at 2.45 pm. He was a current smoker, denied recreational drug use, and had a past medical history of hypertension with poor medicines compliance.

Examination

He was alert and orientated, with a GCS of 15/15. Pulse was 60 beats per minute and regular. BP 158/82 mmHg, heart sounds were normal, chest clear. He had a left sided facial droop with forehead sparing, along with moderate pyramidal weakness of the left arm and leg. His plantar reflex was extensor on the left side, down-going on the right. There was neglect, eye deviation and hemianopia to the left hand side.

V. Wykes, MB, PhD, MRCS • J.P. Grieve, MD, FRCS(SN) (✉)
Department of Neurosurgery, National Hospital for Neurology and Neurosurgery,
London, UK
e-mail: joan.grieve@uclh.nhs.uk

D. Epstein, MBCHB, MRCP
Stroke Medicine, Barnet Hospital, Barnet Hertfordshire, UK

© Springer-Verlag London 2015
S.K. Gill et al. (eds.), *Stroke Medicine: Case Studies from Queen Square*,
DOI 10.1007/978-1-4471-6705-1_12

Investigations

An urgent CT head showed a segment of thrombus within the right MCA (Fig. 12.1a). 12-lead ECG revealed normal sinus rhythm. Routine bloods including glucose, ESR and CRP were within normal limits.

Based on the history, examination and brain imaging, a diagnosis of right MCA occlusion was made. The clinical syndrome was extensive as in addition to the hemiparesis the eye deviation, neglect and hemianopia suggest a "front to back" MCA syndrome. He was thrombolysed with alteplase (0.9 mg/kg) at 2 hours and twenty minutes after symptom onset, and was subsequently transferred to the stroke unit for close physiological monitoring. The neurosurgeons were alerted as the patient was at risk of deterioration which such a large stroke syndrome. Sixteen hours into the admission, the patient's GCS dropped to 11 (E3V3M5). An urgent repeat CT head was arranged, which showed an evolving large right MCA infarct, with cerebral swelling, causing slight midline shift of >5 mm and sulcal effacement (Fig. 12.1b).

The patient was referred urgently to the neurosurgical team and was transferred straight to theatre for a decompressive hemicraniectomy (DHC) to reduce intracranial pressure (ICP) and prevent fatal brain herniation. Blood products were administered, in conjunction with haematology advice in view of recent thrombolysis therapy. The surgery was uncomplicated, and following a period of time on the neurosurgical high dependency unit, he was transferred for rehabilitation. Six months later a titanium cranioplasty was performed to restore skull integrity.

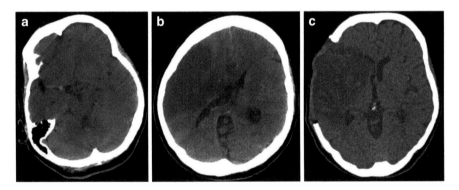

Fig. 12.1 Temporal evolution of right middle cerebral artery territory infarct. (**a**) CT head 2 hours after onset demonstrating hyperdense thrombus in the right MCA (**b**) 16 hours post thrombolysis: CT head demonstrates >50% right MCA territory infarct, midline shift to left >5 mm and sulcal effacement. (**c**) Post emergency decompressive craniectomy: Resolution of midline shift, prominent brain sulci, and infarcted brain herniation through hemicraniectomy site

Discussion

The term malignant middle cerebral artery syndrome (MMCAS) describes the space occupying swelling that follows from a large MCA territory infarct. MMCAS occurs in about 10% of all patients with supratentorial ischaemic stroke, occurring typically between day 2–5 post initial symptom onset, but may occur within 24 hours [1]. Severe brain swelling causes midline shift, elevation in ICP and brain herniation, and carries a mortality rate of up to 80%.

DHC can effectively reduce ICP, reduce mortality and significantly improve neurological outcomes in selected patients with MMCAS. This procedure involves removing a large bone flap, performing a durotomy as the dura can be as equally constrictive as bone. This allows the brain tissue to herniate outwards through the bone flap and so reducing risk of brainstem compression. Three European prospective randomised trials compared DHC within 48 hours of malignant MCA infarct versus best medical management of raised intracranial pressure in patients aged 18–60 years old (French DECIMAL [2], German DESTINY [3] and Dutch HAMLET [4]; [Table 12.1]). A meta-analysis of these trials suggests that decompressive surgery performed within 48 hours of stroke reduces mortality and increases the number of patients with a favourable functional outcome (modified Rankin Scale of less than 4 [6]). However, the intervention does increase the number of patients who survive with a mRS of 4 (Table 12.2). A summary of the meta-analysis is that you exchange a 70% chance of death for a 50:50 chance of a good (or poor)

Table 12.1 Summary of three randomised European Trials comparing decompressive craniotomy to medical therapy for malignant MCA infarct

	DECIMAL	DESTINY	HAMLET
Randomisation	Surgery compared to medical care	Surgery compared to medical care	Surgery compared to medical care
No. patients	38	32	64
Follow-up	1 year	1 year	1 year
	Primary endpoint: functional outcome at 6 months in survivors	Primary endpoint: Mortality at 1 month	Primary endpoint: functional outcome (mRS score)
	Secondary endpoints: survival at 6 and 12 months, functional outcome at 12 months	Secondary endpoints: functional outcome at 6 and 12 months	Secondary endpoints: case fatality, quality of life, symptoms of depression
No. centers	13	6	6

Taken from Johnson (2011) with permission [5]
DECIMAL decompressive craniectomy in malignant MCA infarction, *DESTINY* decompressive surgery for the treatment of malignant infarction of the MCA, *HAMLET* hemicraniectomy after MCA infarction with life-threatening edema trial, *MCA* middle cerebral artery, *mRS* modified Rankin Scale

Table 12.2 Mortality and functional outcomes at 12 months in the pooled analysis of DECIMAL, DESTINY and HAMLET

Outcomes at 12 months	Surgery (%)	Medical care (%)	Statistical significance
Mortality	22	71	$p < 0.0001$
mRS –4	31	2	$p < 0.0001$
mRS <4	74	23	$p < 0.0001$

Taken from Johnson (2011) with permission [5]
DECIMAL decompressive craniectomy in malignant MCA infarction, *DESTINY* decompressive surgery for the treatment of malignant infarction of the MCA, *HAMLET* hemicraniectomy after MCA infarction with life-threatening edema trial, *mRS* modified Rankin Scale

outcome. There are ongoing controversies regarding the indications, timing and benefit of DHC and much research into how to best predict which large infarcts may become "malignant" and cause raised ICP and herniation.

High NIHSS scores indicate increased severity of stroke and can help stratify patients at risk of MMCAS. Patients with early brain imaging (CT or MRI) demonstrating greater than 50% involvement of the MCA territory are at higher risk of MMCAS. Adjacent anterior cerebral artery or posterior cerebral artery territory involvement are predictors of a poor prognosis. A critical infarct volume of greater than 145 ml on diffusion weighted imaging is also a predictor of MMCAS and is associated with a higher mortality [2].

The decision whether to proceed with DHC in patients older than 60 years should be individualised, taking into account pre-stroke functional and cognitive status, patient's advance directive and family wishes (Fig. 12.2). Previous studies of DHC have focused on outcome in patients <60 years, however meta-analysis has demonstrated that >60 year olds have worse mortality and poorer outcome. DESTINY II was a randomised control trial investigating the efficacy of early DHC in patients >60 years with MMCAS and showed benefit of about half the magnitude with higher mRS scores in survivors [8].

DHC is an emergency neurosurgical procedure and once the decision has been made every effort should be aimed at ensuring the patient is ready for surgery in the shortest possible time. The decision needs to be made early and based on the predictive likelihood of deterioration, and not as a response to rapidly escalating mass effect. The physician needs to be bold and say – this patient will be in trouble tomorrow, we need to act today.

Safe transfer should be made to a neurosurgical unit before deterioration (but GCS ≤8 or poor control of airway requires intubation and sedation prior to transfer). If the patient is within 24 hours of thrombolysis, clotting function, APTT, PT, fibrinogen and platelet count should be corrected prior to surgery in discussion with

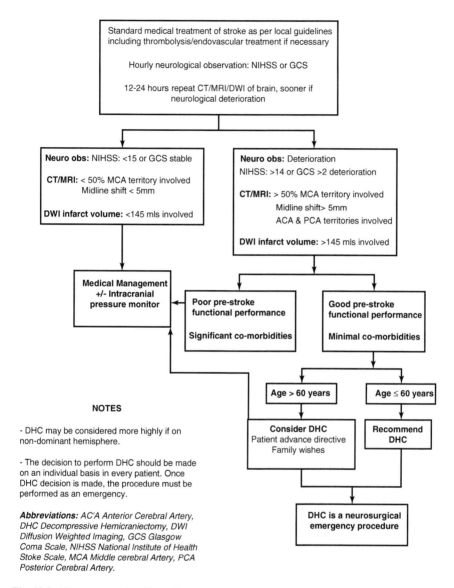

Fig. 12.2   Management algorithm of large MCA stroke (Modified from Wang 2011 [7])

the haematology team. Regular pre-surgical bloods should also be sent. If there are signs suggestive of critically raised ICP (for example anisicoria or dilated pupils), then the procedure has been left too late. Should the patient be deemed not for DHC, best medical management of raised ICP should be commenced. Although the placement of an ICP monitor may help guide medical management, there is controversy as to its validity in MMCAS [9].

Key Clinical Learning Points

1. MMCAS occurs in about 10% of all patients with supratentorial ischaemic stroke, and usually occurs within 48 hours of stroke onset. As a consequence of severe brain swelling there is midline shift, elevation in ICP and brain herniation, carrying a mortality rate of up to 80%
2. Patients at high risk of MMCAS include:

   • Patients with high NIHSS
   • Imaging demonstrating greater than 50% involvement of the MCA territory
   • A critical infarct volume of >145 ml on DWI

3. Patients thought to be at significant risk of MMCAS need to be closely monitored and decisions to operate should be made prospectively
4. MMCAS is a neurosurgical emergency. Decompressive hemicraniectomy must be performed urgently if indicated

Key Radiological Learning Points

Imaging predictors of MMCAS include

1. Early brain imaging (CT or MRI) demonstrating greater than 50% involvement of the MCA territory
2. A critical infarct volume of greater than 145 ml on diffusion weighted imaging
3. Midline shift >5 mm with sulcal effacement

References

1. Qureshi AI, Suarez JI, Yahia AM, et al. Timing of neurologic deterioration in massive middle cerebral artery infarction: a multicenter review. Crit Care Med. 2003;31:272–7.
2. Vahedi K, Vicaut E, Mateo J, et al. Sequential-design, multicenter, randomized, controlled trial of early decompressive craniectomy in malignant middle cerebral artery infarction (DECIMAL Trial). Stroke. 2007;38:2506–17.

3. Jüttler E, Bösel J, Amiri H, et al. Decompressive surgery for the treatment of malignant infarction of the middle cerebral artery II. Stroke. 2011;6:79–86.
4. Hofmeijer J, Kappelle LJ, Algra A, et al. Surgical decompression for space-occupying cerebral infarction (the Hemicraniectomy After Middle Cerebral Artery infarction with Life-threatening Edema Trial [HAMLET]): a multicentre, open, randomised trial. Lancet Neurol. 2009;4:326–33.
5. Johnson RD, Maartens NF, Teddy PJ. Decompressive craniectomy for malignant middle cerebral artery infarction: evidence and controversies. J Clin Neurosci. 2011;18:1018–22.
6. Vahedi K, Hofmeijer J, Jüttler E, et al. Early decompressive surgery in malignant infarction of the middle cerebral artery: a pooled analysis of three randomised controlled trials. Lancet. 2007;6:215–22.
7. Wang DZ, Nair DS, Talkad AV. Acute decompressive hemicraniectomy to control high intracranial pressure in patients with malignant MCA ischaemic strokes. Curr Treat Options Cardiovasc Med. 2011;13:225–32.
8. Jüttler E, Schwab S, Schmiedek P, et al. Decompressive Surgery for the Treatment of Malignant Infarction of the Middle Cerebral Artery (DESTINY): a randomized, controlled trial. Stroke. 2007;9:2518–25.
9. Poca MA, Benejam B, Sahuquillo J, et al. Monitoring intracranial pressure in patients with malignant middle cerebral artery infarction: is this useful? J Neurosurg. 2010;112:648–57.

Chapter 13
A Funny Turn in the Toilet

Sumanjit K. Gill and David Collas

Clinical History

A 56-year-old man presents with non-specific symptoms including some difficult behaviour. He works as a porter and had always been conscientious and popular. He was a life-long smoker and was known to be a moderately heavy drinker, but with no history of alcohol related liver disease. His relatives gave the history. On return from a holiday in Sri Lanka, where he travelled unaccompanied without mishap, he showed some changes in cognition and behaviour, which affected his work. His relatives reported a number of concerns: he had been seen wandering in the rain, standing by a cashpoint at ten at night, and on one occasion failed to recognise his son. After lying lethargic in bed for the whole of one day he was admitted for investigation. History from the patient contributed very little, as he did not perceive any problem. His only past history was hypertension.

Examination

He was cooperative, relaxed and chatty, but dismissive of concerns about his health, and denied that alcohol poses any problem. He was afebrile. Neurological examination of the cranial nerves and peripheral nervous system was normal, but he had brisk reflexes and withdrawal plantar responses. His GCS was 15, but his MTS was impaired at 7/10.

S.K. Gill, BSc Hons, MBBS, MRCP (✉)
Education Unit, National Hospital for Neurology and Neurosurgery,
UCL Institute of Neurology, London, UK
e-mail: sumanjit.gill@nhs.net

D. Collas, BSc, MB, BS FRCP
Stroke Medicine, Watford General Hospital, Watford, UK

© Springer-Verlag London 2015
S.K. Gill et al. (eds.), *Stroke Medicine: Case Studies from Queen Square*,
DOI 10.1007/978-1-4471-6705-1_13

Investigations

Blood tests showed neutrophilia and mild renal impairment – WBC 13.7, urea 14.1, with Hb 15.3, glucose 6.6. A malaria smear was requested. ECG confirmed that he was in sinus rhythm. CT brain showed bilateral areas of low attenuation in the frontal lobes (Fig. 13.1).

Clinical Progress

It was concluded that the lesions explained his changes in behaviour, but the cause of the lesions was not clear. Infarction was dismissed on initial review of the scans as unlikely because of the history, with its gradual onset, and the anatomy because of the bilateral distribution. However, bilateral simultaneous frontal infarcts can arise from a number of mechanisms. They include a relatively common anatomical variants in the anterior circulation in which one anterior cerebral artery supplies both frontal lobes (e.g. bihemispheric A1 segment or 'azygous' A2 segment), venous infarction due to thrombosis of the sagittal sinus, and simultaneous emboli into both anterior cerebral arteries, usually from a cardio-embolic source. However, he was in sinus rhythm and had no signs of infective endocarditis.

Tumours (including "butterfly glioma" or falx meningioma) were considered, but there were no specific imaging features to support these. Cystic glioma and

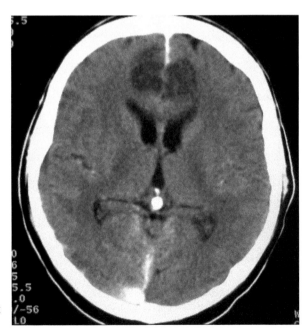

Fig. 13.1 This shows bilateral low density in the medial frontal lobes involving the cingulated gyri

metastasis with predominant oedema remained a possibility. There was no evidence of malignant disease elsewhere. Other possibilities considered included localised infective cerebritis e.g. from fungal infection spreading from frontal sinuses. Tropical infections related to his travel history were explored, but infective screen including malarial smear was negative. Antimicrobial therapy was withheld pending further investigation. CSF examination yielded slightly yellow fluid with a raised WCC of 74 (72 lymphocytes) and a raised RCC of 11,280 in the first bottle and 1,028 in the third bottle. CSF glucose was 3.3 (serum 5.5) and no organisms were seen.

This was inconclusive and a biopsy was considered a possible next step.

However, further neuroradiologist review raised the possibility of vasospasm secondary to subarachnoid haemorrhage (SAH) causing bilateral simultaneous anterior cerebral artery infarcts in both frontal lobes. No subarachnoid blood was demonstrated on the available studies, but this does not exclude recent bleeding.

Further enquiries from sources in Sri Lanka shed more light on the diagnosis. During a night of heavy drinking about 10 days before the current presentation, he had disappeared to an outside toilet. After some time a friend went to look for him and heard a disturbance in the toilet. The apparently very inebriated patient was eventually reached, after breaking the door down. Later reports suggested he had been stiff and frothing at the mouth when discovered in the toilet. He spent a night recovering in hospital recovering before discharge the next day with working diagnosis of a fall in the toilet from intoxication and/or an alcohol induced seizure. He was known to have suffered a fall a few weeks before the holiday. His reported severe headache and neck stiffness were not considered out of the ordinary in the circumstances. It was noteworthy that he still had difficulty walking and needed to be carried to the toilet the day before he flew home, a journey he successfully made unaided.

In retrospect, it seemed likely that the patient suffered a SAH and associated seizure in the toilet in Sri Lanka, and the delay to CT scan explained why no blood was seen. In considering alternative explanations for the CT appearances, the significance of the yellow discolouration of the CSF was overlooked.

A catheter angiogram was performed and showed an anterior communicating aneurysm, confirmed the diagnosis of cerebral infarction in both frontal lobes from vasospasm secondary to SAH from the anterior communicating aneurysm. The aneurysm was secured with detachable endovascular coils.

The subsequent management of this patient centred on neuropsychological evaluation and supported return to work. The behavioural change persisted, with lack of motivation, indifference to requests at times, even if urgent, some resentment of authority and unwillingness to take direction. The patient retained a degree of insight, at least superficially, and agreed to try to modify his behaviour, but in reality this was not carried through and his employment was terminated. His personal relationships suffered from similar difficulties despite his popularity and the willingness of his family and friends to make allowances to persist in supporting him.

Discussion

The diagnosis of SAH is straightforward in cases that present with a classical history of severe, sudden onset headache with associated neck stiffness. However, the diagnosis can be unclear if the presentation is atypical or delayed and the initial symptoms are mild, or if the patient is rendered unconscious with no witnessed history or, as in this case, the symptoms are attributed to other causes. A proportion of patients never report headache and some do not have demonstrable neck stiffness. In cases where there is a delay in presentation, it is important to examine the CSF for breakdown products of haemoglobin [1]. However, more than 2 weeks after the SAH the CSF may be completely normal. In cases where suspicion remains even after negative lumbar puncture, angiography should be considered to look for a cerebral aneurysm.

The imaging appearances of delayed vasospasm after SAH are usually not evident within the first 3 to 4 days after the initial bleed, but can occur from 48 hours onwards [2]. The pathophysiology of arterial vasospasm after SAH is incompletely understood but its severity is influenced by factors including extent of haemorrhage, blood pressure, and intravascular volume [3]. Nimodipine has been shown in a single randomised trial to reduce the incidence of cerebral infarction and improve outcome after SAH [4]. Measuring flow velocities with trans cranial Doppler can be used as a monitoring tool to identify those at risk of developing delayed ischaemic events.

The frontal lobes have a high level of connectivity to deeper brain structures and are implicated in planning, speech production, decision-making, judgment impulse control and memory functions. Damage can range from causing striking disinhibition and inappropriate social behaviours to subtler frontal lobe pathology causing dysexecutive syndromes and inability to make decisions. Tests of frontal lobe function are included in generalised tests of cognitive function such as the ACE-R or MoCA but are more thoroughly assessed in specific tests such as the frontal lobe battery.

Key Clinical Learning Points
1. Marked brain damage in the frontal lobes may be overlooked for some time; the apparent gradual development of symptoms (which is more the gradual realisation that there is something wrong with the patient's behaviour) is an exception to the usual rule that the symptoms of stroke come on suddenly
2. The problems of frontal lobe dysfunction, even though subtle, carry serious consequences for the individual and their family, friends and employers if not taken seriously. Neurological clues on examination might include frontal release signs and primitive reflexes
3. Bilateral infarcts are unusual unless there is a cardiac source, such as AF or infective endocarditis, but other mechanisms should be considered, including cerebral venous thrombosis and vasospasm from SAH
4. SAH can present without a typical history of headache and neck stiffness, especially if the presentation is delayed

Key Radiological Learning Points
1. An angiogram performed in the acute phase of a subarachnoid haemorrhage may fail to reveal an aneurysm because of spasm, pressure from the haematoma, or obscuration by the blood and may need to be performed after an interval

References

1. Liebenberg WA, Worth R, Firth GB, et al. Aneurysmal subarachnoid haemorrhage: guidance in making the correct diagnosis. Postgrad Med J. 2005;81:470–473.
2. Heros RC, Zervas NT, Varsos V. Cerebral vasospasm after subarachnoid haemorrhage: an update. Ann Neurol. 2004;14(6):599–608.
3. Fisher CM, Kistler JP, Davis J. Relation of cerebral vasospasm to subarachnoid haemorrhage visualised by computerised tomographic scanning. Neurosurgery. 1980;6(1):1–9.
4. Pickard JD, Murray GD, Illingworth R, et al. Effect of oral nimodipine on cerebral infarction and outcome after subarachnoid haemorrhage: British aneurysm nimodipine trial. Br Med J. 1989;298(6):36–42.

Chapter 14
A Strategic Infarct Leading to Mild Cognitive Impairment

Sumanjit K. Gill and Alexander Leff

Clinical History

A 59-year-old right-handed male nurse presented to the Accident and Emergency department with a 2-day history of confusion. His wife had noticed that he had quiet speech and that he had not been talking much with her. She described him as being restless throughout the night with incomprehensible mumbling. When he tried to text her, she was unable to read it as the letters were jumbled. He seemed confused and when asked to go shopping for food he returned with two cauliflowers, which she thought odd and prompted her to seek medical attention. He had no vascular risk factors. The only positive family history was that his father had hereditary neuropathy with liability to pressure palsies.

Examination

The patient walked normally into the Accident and Emergency department. Cardiovascular examination was normal except for a high blood pressure. The admitting senior house officer notes that he seemed disorientated and was slow to respond. His affect was blunted. His speech was hypophonic and lacked fluency. The remainder of the neurological examination was normal. The Montreal Cognitive Assessment

S.K. Gill, BSc.hons, MBBS, MRCP (✉)
Education Unit, National Hospital for Neurology and Neurosurgery,
UCL Institute of Neurology, London, UK
e-mail: sumanjit.gill@nhs.net

A. Leff, PhD, FRCP
Institute of Cognitive Neuroscience and Department of Brain Repair and Rehabilitation,
UCL Institute of Neurology, University College London and National Hospital
for Neurology and Neurosurgery, London, UK
e-mail: a.leff@ucl.ac.uk

© Springer-Verlag London 2015
S.K. Gill et al. (eds.), *Stroke Medicine: Case Studies from Queen Square*,
DOI 10.1007/978-1-4471-6705-1_14

Table 14.1 MoCA assessment at 2 days and 6 weeks post stroke. This demonstrates a deficit in verbal short-term memory which did not resolve

DOMAIN	Visuo spatial	Naming	Repetition	Attention	Language	Abstraction	Delayed recall	Orientation
2 days post stroke	4/5	3/3	2/2	5/6	2/3 lexical fluency	1/2 conceptualisation	0/5	5/6 date
6 weeks post stroke	n/a	n/a	2	5/5	3	2/2	0/5	6/6

(MoCA) was carried out (See Table 14.1.). This showed that he was orientated in time, place and person and that the confusion was the result of aphasia.

Investigations

CT brain was normal. MRI done the day after his admission showed an acute infarct in the left thalamus (Figs. 14.1 and 14.2).

Clinical Progress

A diagnosis was made of dysphasia secondary to an acute thalamic infarct. No cause was identified. On review 6 weeks after onset, he described a persisting anomia and memory problems. His verbal fluency had improved and he did not describe any persisting language deficit tests. A MoCA was completed over the telephone, which demonstrated a persisting deficit (Table 14.1).

Discussion

This case demonstrates that a strategic placed single small subcortical infarct can lead to significant cognitive impairment, in this case dysphasia resulting from a thalamic infarct. It is quite possible that a more detailed cognitive assessment by a

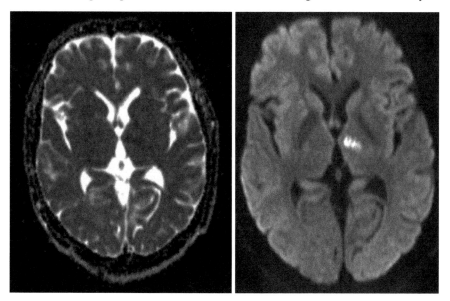

Fig. 14.1 MRI with ADC map (*left figure*) and DWI (*right figure*) showing an acute infarct in the left thalamus

Fig. 14.2 MRI T1 weighted
fluid attenuated image,
coronal slice, showing the
infarct in the left thalamus

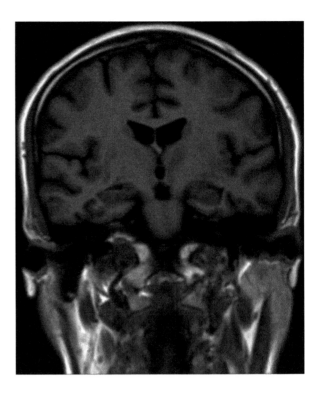

neuropsychologist would have revealed other more subtle defects in cognitive function, given that the MoCA is only a screening tool and is not intended to be diagnostic [1].

More extensive cognitive impairment can arise from such strategic placed infarcts particularly if they are bilateral e.g. when bilateral thalamic infarction occurs as a result of occlusion of a normal anatomical variant artery in which a single common perforating branch of the tip of the basilar artery supplies both thalami. Such strategic thalamic infarcts are recognized to cause of up to 5% of cases of vascular dementia [2].

The thalamus exerts its influence on emotional processing and memory via cortical projections to the cingulate gyrus and through its association with the hypothalamus. Infarcts in the tuberothalamic and paramedian nuclei are more likely to be associated with language deficits with paramedian lesions causing more prominent neuropsychiatric features. Infarcts in the anterior thalamus are due to occlusion of the polar artery, a branch of the posterior communicating artery, and typically cause neuropsychological symptoms and behavioural change. Infarcts of the thalamic nuclei can present with aphasia, amnesia and executive dysfunction. Although left-sided infarcts were thought more likely to cause language symptoms and right-sided infarcts to cause visuospatial problems, a recent series found no such association [3].

Post-stroke aphasia is common occurring in up 30% of stroke patients [4], typically those with left hemispheric lesions. This case demonstrates how language and cognitive deficits often occur in combination. Aphasia usually occurs as a result of an infarct or haemorrhage in the anterior circulation from disruption to the perisylvian language centres. Typical patterns of impairment are shown in Table 14.2. It is

Table 14.2 Patterns of aphasia [12]

	Broca's	Wernicke's	Conduction	Transcortical Broca's	Transcortical Wernickes
Description	Non fluent aphasia, effortful speech	Fluent aphasia	Fluent aphasia	Unable to produce spontaneous speech	Fluent aphasia
Naming	impaired	impaired	intact	impaired	intact
Repetition	impaired	impaired	impaired	intact	intact
Comprehension	intact	impaired	intact	intact	impaired

not entirely clear how subcortical infarcts cause aphasia. A reasonable hypothesis is that both cortico-thalamic and thalamo-cortical connections are damaged, affecting hierarchical processing of language.

There is clear evidence for the efficacy of speech and language therapy in treating post-stroke aphasia based intensity of treatment. A significant treatment effect was seen when patients were given at least 8 hours a week of therapy [5], which is difficult to achieve in an standard rehabilitation unit setting where resources will not provide for this. In terms of pharmacotherapy, dopamine agonists have been explored as an as an adjunct to speech and language therapy, but there is only weak evidence for a positive effect [6]. Memantine and donepezil have been shown to have possible benefits in shown in initial studies [7, 8].

Post-stroke cognitive impairment is found in up to 10% of patients after their first ever stroke and more than 30% after recurrent stroke [9]. The main predictors of cognitive impairment after stroke identified in a meta-analysis of 73 studies, were older age, female sex, lower educational attainment, diabetes, and atrial fibrillation. Others included left hemisphere involvement, presence of dysphasia and recurrent strokes. Early recognition is vital to guide the rehabilitation process and to inform discharge planning. The MoCA is a widely available test of cognitive function that has been shown to be more sensitive at detecting post stroke cognitive deficits that the MMSE [10]. The gold standard remains a neuropsychological battery but lack of funding for psychologists to administer and interpret the tests remains a barrier to achieving routine detailed neuropsychological testing in the majority of units [11].

Key Clinical Learning Points
- Cognitive deficits can occur secondary to strokes in areas of the brain not classically associated with cognitive function e.g. the thalamus
- The MoCA can be used to assess cognitive function across a variety of domains
- Cognitive deficits can be subtle with a high impact on functional ability, and the clinician should be aware of the possibility of their existence in the absence of overt confusion
- Language deficits are often a component of cognitive impairment and should be treated with high intensity speech and language therapy

References

1. Pendlebury ST, Welch SJ, Cuthburtson FC, et al. Telephone assessment of cognitive function after transient ischaemic attack and stroke: modified telephone interview of cognitive status and telephone montreal cognitive assessment versus face-to-face montreal cognitive assessment and neuropsychological battery. Stroke. 2013;44(1):227–9.
2. Szirmai I, Vastagh I, Szombathelyi E, et al. Strategic infarcts of the thalamus in vascular dementia. J Neurol Sci. 2002;203–4:91–7.
3. Tanaka H, Hoshino Y, Watanabe Y, et al. A Case of Strategic Infarct Mild Cognitive Impairment. Neurologist. 2012;18(4):211–13.
4. Engelter ST, Gostynski M, Papa S, et al. Epidemiology of aphasia attributable to first ever stroke. Stroke. 2006;37:1379–84.
5. Bhogal SK, Teasell R, Speechley M. Intensity of aphasia therapy impact on recovery. Stroke. 2003;34:987–93.
6. Gill SK, Leff A. Dopaminergic therapy in aphasia. Aphasiology. 2013;28(2):155–70. doi:10.1080/02687038.2013.802286.
7. Berthier ML, Green C, Lara JP, et al. Memantine and constraint induced aphasia therapy in chronic post stroke aphasia. Ann Neurol. 2009;65:577–85. doi:10.1002/ana.21597.
8. Berthier ML, Hinojosa J, del Carmen MM, et al. Open label study of donepezil in chronic post stroke aphasia. Neurology. 2003;60(7):1218–9.
9. Pendlebury S, Rothwell PM. Prevalence, incidence and factors associated with pre stroke and post stroke dementia: a systematic review and metanalysis. Lancet Neurol. 2009;8:1006–18.
10. Pendlebury ST, Mariz J, Bull L, et al. MoCA, ACE-R and MMSE versus the national institute of neurological disorders and stroke-Canadian network vascular cognitive impairment harmonisation standards neuropsychological battery after TIA and stroke. Stroke. 2012;43: 464–9.
11. Chan E, Khan S, Oliver R, et al. Underestimation of cognitive impairments by the Montreal Cognitive Assessment (MoCA): a Study in Subacute Stroke. Journal of the Neurological Sciences. 2014;343(1–2). doi:10.1016/j.jns.2014.05.005.
12. Croquelois A, Godefroy O. Aphasic, arthric, calculation and auditory disorders. In: Godefroy O, editor. The behavioural and cognitive neurology of stroke. Secondth ed. Cambridge: Cambridge University Press; 2013. p. 65–75.

Chapter 15
A Misbehaving Limb

Menelaos Pipis and Sumanjit K. Gill

Clinical History

An 87-year-old right-handed woman was brought to the Emergency Department after a fall at home. She walked with the assistance of a frame, but lost her balance, falling to the right side. She denied any head injury or loss of consciousness, and did not recall having any palpitations, postural symptoms or chest pain. However, she reported that since the fall, she had noticed her left arm was constantly moving in an uncontrollable fashion.

Her past medical history included long-standing epilepsy, which was well controlled, congestive cardiac failure, hypertension and hypercholesterolaemia. There was no known family history of abnormal limb movements or chorea. She was a non-smoker, seldom drank alcohol and was independent in activities of daily living.

Examination

She looked well and was alert with an abbreviated mental test score (AMTS) of 10 out of 10. On general inspection, there were continuous writhing movements of the left arm and left orofacial muscles. Otherwise neurological examination was normal. Her cardiovascular examination revealed an irregularly irregular pulse with normal heart sounds. Physical examination of the abdominal and respiratory systems as well as the skin and joints was unremarkable.

M. Pipis, MBBS, BSc (Hons), MRCP
Department of Medicine, Northwick Park Hospital, Harrow, Middlesex, London, UK

S.K. Gill, BSc Hons, MBBS, MRCP (✉)
Education Unit, National Hospital for Neurology and Neurosurgery,
UCL Institute of Neurology, London, UK
e-mail: sumanjit.gill@nhs.net

© Springer-Verlag London 2015
S.K. Gill et al. (eds.), *Stroke Medicine: Case Studies from Queen Square*,
DOI 10.1007/978-1-4471-6705-1_15

Investigations

At the time of admission, routine blood tests including full blood count, renal and thyroid function, clotting screen, C-reactive protein, fasting glucose, cholesterol and triglycerides were within normal ranges. The patient's ECG showed atrial fibrillation at a rate of 87 bpm. Her CT head scan showed no evidence of an acute haemorrhage or infarct, but revealed bilateral extensive leukoaraiosis suggestive of small vessel ischaemic damage in a periventricular and deep distribution.

A MRI scan of the brain with diffusion weighted images was taken and is shown below (Figs. 15.1 and 15.2):

The patient was diagnosed with an acute right thalamic infarct, likely embolic in nature and secondary to atrial fibrillation. She was started on oral anticoagulation with a direct thrombin inhibitor (dabigatran). Her continuous, ballistic movements were quickly and well controlled with the initiation of tetrabenazine 25 mg once daily, subsequently increased to 25 mg twice daily. She continued to improve and was able to ambulate with the aid of her walking frame by discharge. Four months after her initial presentation her choreiform movements had completely resolved.

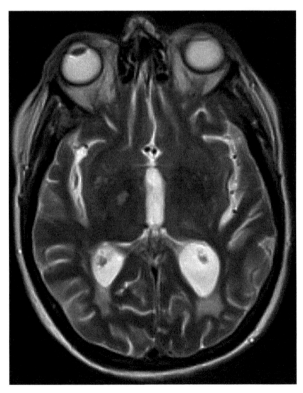

Fig. 15.1 T2 weighted image shows a lesion in the right ventro-lateral thalamus

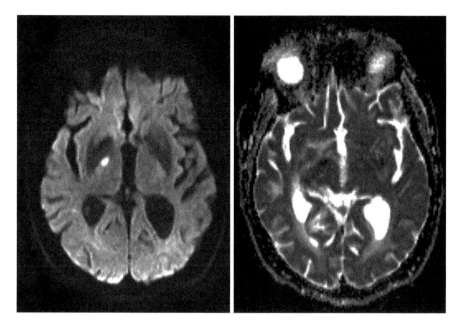

Fig. 15.2 DWI (*left*) and ADC map (*right*) demonstrating a matched defect in the right thalamus

Discussion

The basal ganglia have a pivotal role in the production of context-dependent motor behaviours. Converging data from the fields of neuroanatomy, neuropharmacology and pathophysiology have led to concurring hypotheses regarding their functional organization in health and disease. The 'input nuclei' consist of the caudate nucleus and putamen (collectively known as the striatum) and receive the majority of afferents from the cortical mantle, in a highly topographical manner. The processing of cortical information within the basal ganglia is integrated with inputs from various other brain structures including the intralaminar thalamic nuclei, which primarily innervate the striatum [1] (Fig. 15.3).

This processed information is transmitted via two routes, to the medial segment of the globus pallidus and the pars reticulata of the substantia nigra. Together, these two homologous structures are regarded as the 'output' section of the basal ganglia from which the majority of efferent fibres originate and project to other levels of the neuraxis. These projections primarily relay to the ventral thalamus and ultimately reach the cerebral cortex and more specifically the supplementary motor area [1].

The role of the basal ganglia is more easily understood if one studies the clinical manifestations of neurological disorders of the basal ganglia. Strategic lesions of the basal ganglia and occasionally other brain structures, which may be vascular, structural, infective, traumatic or hypoxic in origin, can all result in secondary movement disorders [2]. However, movement disorders of a vascular origin differ in their clinical presentation, natural history, prognosis and treatment. Haemorrhagic

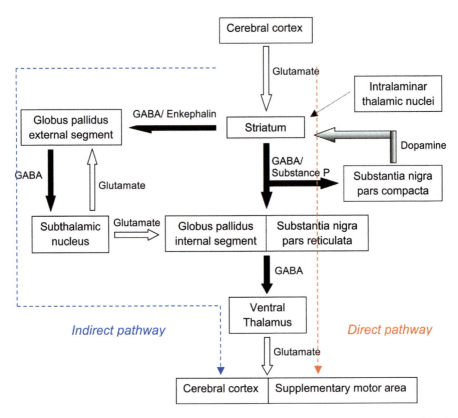

Fig. 15.3 A basic model of the synaptic organisation of the basal ganglia with a representation of the direct and indirect pathways. The *white-filled arrows* indicate excitatory neurotransmission and the *dark-filled arrows* indicate inhibitory neurotransmission

or ischaemic strokes may account for approximately 25% of secondary movement disorders and can occur immediately after a stroke or have a delayed presentation. In fact, the latency between an acute stroke and the onset of a movement disorder may vary from less than a day to several years after the acute vascular insult [2, 3]. Nonetheless, hyperkinetic or hypokinetic (parkinsonism) movement disorders are uncommon after stroke. In the Lausanne stroke registry, of 2,500 cases of first stroke, 1% of patients suffered from an acute or delayed hyperkinetic movement disorder [4]. Most cases involved lesions in the territories of the middle and posterior cerebral arteries and hemiballismus and hemichorea were the commonest movement disorders (4 out of 10) reported to occur after a stroke. Hemidystonia, stereotypias, jerky dystonia, myoclonus, asterixis and tremor were some of the other secondary movement disorders observed in the study's cohort and 90% of these resolved within 6 months.

Ballismus and Chorea

Hemiballismus is an abnormal, involuntary, poorly-predictable movement that usually involves the arm and leg on one side of the body. It can also be associated with mandibular, orobuccal, lingual and dystonic movements. It is contorting and continuous and of a rotatory nature. In contrast, chorea is characterised by more subtle, low-amplitude, brief and non-repetitive movements that appear to spread from one muscle to the next. Following stroke, chorea may be associated with mild sensory disturbances and motor weakness and is frequently accompanied by athetosis [2, 3].

Whilst ballismus after stroke is rare, cerebrovascular disease has been reported to be its commonest cause [3]. Even though a vascular lesion affecting the contralateral subthalamic nucleus is the most consistent neuropathological finding in patients with hemiballismus, lesions in the thalamus, caudate nucleus and putamen can also be associated with this hyperkinetic disorder [2, 3]. In our case, a thalamic infarct was responsible for producing ballistic movements in the contralateral side of the body. Bearing in mind that the net output signal of the basal ganglia to the thalamus under resting conditions is one of inhibition [1], it may be difficult to explain how a dysregulation in the thalamus, which is the 'receiver' of the basal ganglia efferents, would lead to a disinhibition and hence a hyperkinetic disorder. However, a plausible neuronal link justifying this correlation, may lie in the modulatory afferents that the striatum receives from the intralaminar thalamic nuclei. A thalamic lesion that dysregulates these modulators may in turn influence the processing of cortical information within the basal ganglia in such a way that results in hyperkinesis and ballismus.

Most patients with new onset hemiballismus and hemichorea, tend to develop these disorders immediately after or within a few days of a stroke. Frequently, patients that develop hemiballismus witness their ballistic movements to become less severe with time, evolve into hemichorea and later to hemidystonia [2, 3]. The observation of new onset chorea in the context of an acute stroke should prompt the physician to exclude a diagnosis of hyperglycaemic chorea and additionally consider and investigate for an underlying vasculitis (such as systemic lupus erythematosus), hyperviscocity disorder (such as paraproteinaemia) or coagulopathy (such as antiphospholipid syndrome) [3]. Studies have shown evidence that hemiballismus follows a benign course with a spontaneous recovery in up to a quarter of cases and an associated survival rate of up to 88% after 3 years [3].

Ballismus and chorea tend to respond to similar pharmacological therapies. The most commonly reported effective agents include dopamine receptor antagonists (such as a haloperidol), benzodiazepines (such as diazepam and clonazepam), tetrabenazine (which was used in our case), topiramate, sodium valproate and even local intramascular injections of botulinum toxin [2, 3].

Dystonia

Dystonia refers to involuntary and sustained muscle contractions which usually result in abnormal postures or repetitive twisting movements [2]. It was the second commonest movement disorder observed in the Lausanne stroke registry [4], and unlike hemiballismus, evidence shows it to have a delayed onset after stroke by an average of 9.5 months [3]. Another variant of stroke-related dystonia is dystonic myoclonus, a disorder which has been described as a 'jerky dystonic unsteady hand' [2]. Apart from lesions of the putamen (commonest site), dystonia has also been attributed to lesions of the thalamus, caudate nucleus, globus pallidus and midbrain.

Unfortunately, dystonia after cerebrovascular disease shows a poor response to pharmacological therapy. Even though some benefit has been reported from the use of anticholinergics, dopamine receptor antagonists, baclofen and benzo-diazepines, probably the best medical approach are local intramascular injec-tions of botulinum toxin, especially in cases of focal and functionally disabling dystonia [2, 3].

Myoclonus and Asterixis

Myoclonus consists of brief and involuntary twitching of a muscle or muscle groups and after stroke can affect the upper and lower limbs, the voice, and less frequently, the face. Other than in the basal ganglia, lesions in the thalamus, frontoparietal lobes, midbrain and pons have been associated with post-stroke myoclonus [2, 3]. Asterixis consists of poorly-predictable interruptions of sustained voluntary muscle contraction thus resulting in brief losses of posture. Following stroke, it has been attributed to lesions in various brain regions such as the thalamus, frontal lobe, mid-brain and cerebellum [2, 3].

Treatment for post-stroke myoclonus with clonazepam and sodium valproate is usually only indicated when the abnormal movements interfere with activities and function. Asterixis is usually self-limited and does not require medical treat-ment [2].

Tremor and Tics

Holmes' tremor is another movement disorder that has been described to occur after stroke. It is a resting tremor, which is irregular and of low frequency, tends to involve the upper limbs and worsens with goal-orientated movements [2]. It com-monly results from lesions in the brainstem, as well as the thalamus and cerebellum, thus highlighting the probable involvement of the nigrostiatal pathways in its pathophysiology. Post-stroke tremor is usually refractory to medical treatment but dopaminergic pharmacotherapies such as levodopa, as well as propranolol, clonazepam, valproic acid and levetiracetam have been reported to offer symptomatic relief [3]. When response to oral medications is poor, surgical intervention such as thalamic deep brain stimulation and ventrointermedius thalamotomy may be required [2, 3].

Tics are characterised by brief and involuntary motor twitches or sounds (phonic tics). Isolated reports have described them to occur after strokes in the basal ganglia and, if needed, can be treated with alpha-receptor agonists, such as clonidine or dopamine receptor antagonists such as risperidone [3].

Vascular Parkinsonism

"Vascular parkinsonism" is the main hypokinetic movement disorder observed after cerebrovascular disease, and it encompasses a heterogeneous group of conditions with features that resemble Parkinson's Disease. Even though acute onset of parkinsonism can be attributed to strokes in the midbrain and basal ganglia, it is now recognised that people with chronic small vessel cerebrovascular disease can also develop a progressive condition characterised by parkinsonian features [2, 3]. The Lausanne stroke study only included patients with hyperkinetic post-stroke movement disorders, but in a study from Ecuador that evaluated 56 patients (out of 1,500) with post-stroke involuntary abnormal movements, 11% of patients had developed parkinsonism [5]. In this study, the average latency between diagnosis of the stroke and the onset of parkinsonism was 117.5 days and it was the longest time interval when compared to that of other post-stroke movement disorders.

The classical form of vascular parkinsonism presents as 'lower body parkinsonism', with rigidity and bradykinesia that predominantly affects the legs and spares the arms. It is characterised by gait abnormality: either unstable broad-based or marche a petit pas, shuffling and often freezing gait, postural instability and gait ignition failure [2]. Resting tremor is not typical, and if present it is usually mild. This condition can be associated with pyramidal signs, as well as pseudobulbar palsy, incontinence, dementia, hypertension and diabetes [2]. The syndrome is more accurately termed gait apraxia when examination on the couch is often unremarkable, though functional movement of the legs is very impaired and is a major cause of falls in the elderly.

Conventional dopaminergic therapy may improve symptoms in approximately one third to half of patients with vascular parkinsonism, but the effects are usually short-lived [2, 3]. The mainstay of management should include physiotherapy and occupational therapy, along with treatment of hypertension, diabetes and other vascular risk factors.

Conclusion

The prevalence of movement disorders after stroke is small and they have a tendency to resolve over time. Nonetheless, the disability and adverse long-term outcomes (financial, psychological and social) that may accompany them, as well as the availability of appropriate therapy, necessitates their early recognition and management. When they occur as a late manifestation of an acute stroke, a raised awareness and clinical suspicion, will aid in their early recognition and management.

Key Clinical Learning Points
1. Movement disorders following stroke are uncommon and have a tendency to resolve
2. Secondary movement disorders and can occur immediately after a stroke or have a delayed presentation
3. Stroke-related movement disorders can adversely affect rehabilitation and long-term morbidity if not recognised and managed appropriately

Key Radiological Learning Points
1. Lesions giving rise to movement disorders need not be in the basal ganglia; lesions in other brain regions have been reported
2. Diffusion weighted imaging may be required to demonstrate a small lesion that correlates with the clinical presentation, especially if there is background cerebrovascular ischaemic damage

References

1. Bolam JP, Hanley JJ, Booth PAC, et al. Synaptic organisation of the basal ganglia. J Anat. 2000;196:527–42.
2. Mehanna R, Jankovic J. Movement disorders in cerebrovascular disease. Lancet Neurol. 2013;12:597–608.
3. Bansil S, Prakash N, Kaye J, et al. Movement disorders after stroke in adults: a review. Tremor Other Hyperkinet Mov. 2012;2: tre-02-42-195-1.
4. Ghika-Schmid F, Ghika J, Regli F, et al. Hyperkinetic movement disorders during and after acute stroke: the Lausanne Stroke Registry. J Neurol Sci. 1997;146:109–16.
5. Alarcon F, Zijlmans JCM, Duenas G, et al. Post-stroke movement disorders: report of 56 patients. J Neurol Neurosurg Psychiatry. 2004;75:1568–74.

Chapter 16
More Than Just a Sore Throat

Sumanjit K. Gill and David Collas

Clinical History

A 22-year-old female university student visited her GP with a history of a sore throat for 1 week. She was given antibiotics but did not take them, reasoning that the cause was likely to be viral. Over the next week she became tired and feverish, with headache and swelling of her left eye. She was then brought home from her halls of residence by her parents, and presented to the Accident and Emergency department of her local hospital. She has no past medical history, but reveals that she took the "morning-after pill" (post-coital contraception) a week earlier.

Examination

She was alert when first seen, but was febrile (temperature 38.8 °C) with mild neck stiffness, cervical lymphadenopathy and left parotid gland swelling. There was proptosis and chemosis of the left eye, with yellow discharge from the eye; there was no neurological deficit except a partial ophthalmoplegia of the left eye. There was no rash and she was haemodynamically stable.

S.K. Gill, BSc Hons, MBBS, MRCP (✉)
Education Unit, National Hospital for Neurology and Neurosurgery,
UCL Institute of Neurology, London, UK
e-mail: sumanjit.gill@nhs.net

D. Collas, BSc, MB, BS FRCP
Stroke Medicine, Watford General Hospital, Watford, UK

© Springer-Verlag London 2015
S.K. Gill et al. (eds.), *Stroke Medicine: Case Studies from Queen Square*,
DOI 10.1007/978-1-4471-6705-1_16

103

Investigations

An admission chest X-ray showed patches of consolidation, some with cavity formation. CT thorax confirmed bilateral patchy cavitating lesions (Fig. 16.1). It also showed a tonsillar abscess constricting the oropharynx, enhancing cervical lymph nodes and parotid gland swelling. Laboratory investigations showed a marked inflammatory response with a CRP of 302, leukocytosis (WCC 22×10^{-9} L) and thrombocytopaenia. She also had a prolonged prothrombin time of 15.3 s and an elevated alanine aminotransferase of 169 units/L.

Clinical Progress

Although stable, she was transferred to ITU for respiratory monitoring. Suggested diagnoses include glandular fever, toxic shock syndrome, cavitating pneumonia (*Staphylococcus* or *Klebsiella*), meningitis (including TB in view of the cavitating lung lesions) and cavernous sinus thrombosis because of her proptosis. From the start, an additional diagnosis of Lemierre's syndrome was also entertained. Swabs and cultures were taken and a CT brain requested.

The CT showed normal brain with an "incidental note" made of mild left maxillary, left sphenoid and ethmoid sinusitis, and thickening of the soft tissues was seen in the region of the left parotid gland and the left temporalis muscle, indicative of possible inflammation. Oedema of the upper eyelid and subcutaneous tissues was also noted but the eyeballs were symmetrical, with no evidence of any retrobulbar inflammation, mass lesion or intracranial collection.

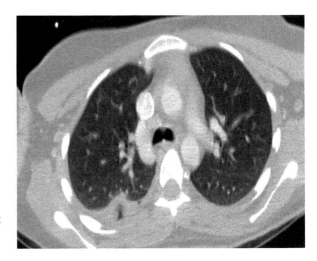

Fig. 16.1 CT chest showing cavitating areas of consolidation

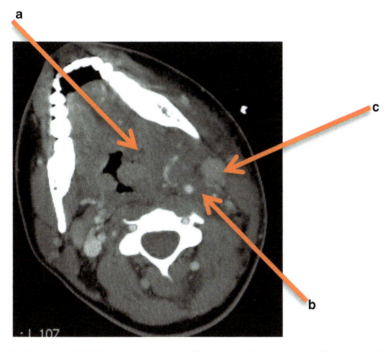

Fig. 16.2 Her second CT head showing a tonsillar abscess (**a**), an occluded left internal jugular vein (**b**) and an enlarged lymph node (**c**)

The decision was taken to start anticoagulants, but haematological advice was to delay this until she had received a platelet transfusion.

After 3 days on antibiotics in the face of negative cultures from throat swabs, urine and blood (there was no sputum), she deteriorated and was noted to have increased proptosis, some restriction of eye movement, possible involvement of the right eye and increasing drowsiness. The CT brain was repeated. This showed occlusion of the left jugular vein, and concurrent cavernous sinus thrombus, with a tonsillar abscess and enlarged enhancing tonsillar lymph node (Fig. 16.2). There was no venous sinus thrombosis outside the cavernous sinus. The diagnosis of Lemierre's syndrome was now considered the most likely.

Despite further changes in her multiple antibiotic regimen, she became obtunded with increasing proptosis, a fixed left pupil, papilloedema and haemodynamic insta-bility. Both carotid arteries were now narrowed, either by in situ thrombosis caused by the presumed bacterial infection despite heparin, spasm or by external compres-sion from local swelling and inflammation (Fig. 16.3). This led to bilateral hypoxic brain damage and massive bi-hemispheric infarction culminating in death 5 days after her initial presentation (Fig. 16.4).

Autopsy showed pus in both cavernous sinus and in bilaterally thrombosed jugular veins.

Fig. 16.3 The left carotid is
compromised by local
swelling

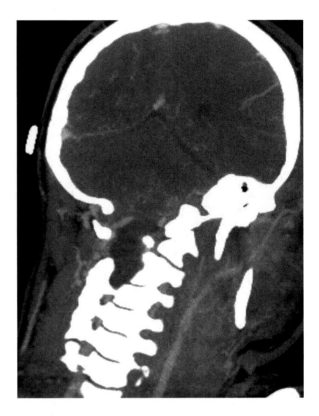

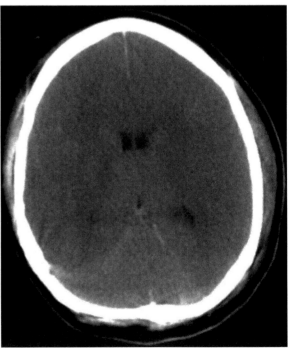

Fig. 16.4 Bilateral cerebral
oedema due to bilateral
hemisphere infarction

Discussion

Lemierre's syndrome, first described in 1936, is a rare, potentially lethal complication of oropharyngeal sepsis [1]. It occurs when *Fusobacterium necrophorum*, a normal part of oral flora, becomes invasive and propagates proximally with septic emboli to the lungs, retrogradely causing cavernous thrombosis and locally into the carotid sheath. This leads to raised intracranial pressure from venous thrombosis and venous infarction or diffuse ischaemia, with potentially devastating consequences. Increased awareness of this once common condition, which became increasingly rare after the introduction and widespread use of antibiotics and now largely forgotten and overlooked, is essential if fatal outcomes, such as occurred in this case, are to be avoided. It is to be hoped that improving awareness and prompt use of antibiotics and anticoagulation (though lacking grade 1 evidence) will help achieve a better outcome.

Key Clinical Learning Points
1. A sore throat, whilst one of the most common reasons for presentation to a general practitioner, can lead to serious complications, but patients may not appreciate this and fail to take antibiotics even in those cases where they are prescribed
2. Cavitating pneumonia may be due to septic emboli as well as more familiar lung pathogens associated with cavitation as a primary phenomenon (i.e. *Staphylococcus*, *Klebsiella*, TB). Sources for these emboli may include the pharynx via the internal jugular vein
3. Appropriate antibiotics and anticoagulation are urgently indicated once Lemierre's syndrome is suspected but may still fail to prevent progression
4. Microbiology tests may fail to yield an organism despite multiple samples, and antibiotic treatment may need to be changed or added to on empirical grounds, following the advice of the microbiologist

Key Radiological Learning Points
1. Careful inspection of all aspects of an X-ray, such as detection of tonsillar swelling and air (signs of abscess), soft tissue swelling (parotid), and sinusitis, and crucially noticing jugular abnormalities on a contrast scan, will assist diagnosis, particularly if they are interpreted with all the clinical information
2. Repeating scans is crucial if patient's condition deteriorates despite active treatment

Reference

1. Lemierre A. On certain septicaemias due to anaerobic organisms. Lancet. 1936;1:701–3.

Chapter 17
An MRI Saves a Patient from Unnecessary Surgery

Anne Jutta Schmitt and Robert Simister

Clinical History

A 58-year-old right-handed male Italian tourist presented to the emergency department with a history of transient left arm and leg weakness of abrupt onset and associated with slurred speech. The weakness occurred whilst travelling on the train to London. He gave a history of a similar event occurring in Italy 6 weeks earlier, when he was told that a narrowing of the right carotid artery that might require surgery. He also gave a history of hypertension, diabetes mellitus and hypercholesterolaemia and he smoked cigarettes. He described symptoms of intermittent claudication in both legs suggesting peripheral vascular disease. At the time of presentation he was taking aspirin, ezetemibe and doxazosin.

Examination

On examination he was alert and orientated. There was minimal dysarthria but otherwise he was thought to be neurologically intact. His blood pressure was elevated at 151/85 mmHg but his heart sounds were normal and his pulse was regular.

A.J. Schmitt, Dr. Med. Univ.
Department of Radiology, University College London Hospital,
London, UK
e-mail: nnschmitt@gmail.com

R. Simister, MA, FRCP, PhD (✉)
Comprehensive Stroke Service, National Hospital for
Neurology and Neurosurgery, UCLH Trust, London, UK
e-mail: robert.simister@uclh.nhs.uk

© Springer-Verlag London 2015
S.K. Gill et al. (eds.), *Stroke Medicine: Case Studies from Queen Square*,
DOI 10.1007/978-1-4471-6705-1_17

Investigations

Routine blood tests show elevated cholesterol but were otherwise normal. His 12 lead ECG revealed only a sinus bradycardia.

Initial imaging with a CT head and CTA of the extracranial and intracranial arteries showed an established focus of low attenuation in the left thalamus and widespread atheromatous arteriopathy, most marked at the right carotid bifurcation with a calcified plaque at the left vertebral artery origin causing mild stenosis and mild stenosis of the mid portion of the basilar artery. There was no visible acute infarction. A carotid Doppler ultrasound showed ulcerated soft plaque and a 60–69% stenosis at the origin of the right internal carotid artery.

An MRI with vascular sequences revealed a small acute infarct with restricted diffusion in the right side of the pons at the level of the inferior cerebellar peduncles. Small established infarcts were seen in the left thalamus. Interestingly, no lesion could be identified in the right anterior circulation that might have explained the earlier event attributed in Italy to a symptomatic right ICA plaque. The MRA demonstrated the previously identified right ICA significant stenosis and demonstrated that the mid segment basilar artery narrowing was at the level of the pontine perforator artery territory acute infarct (Figs. 17.1 and 17.2).

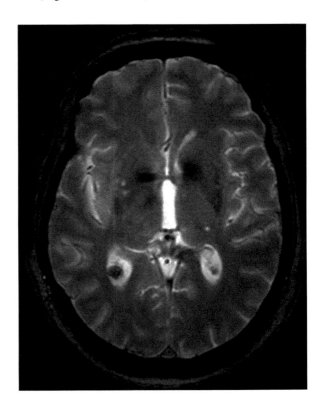

Fig. 17.1 T2 weighted imaging showing a tiny mature left thalamic infarct only

Fig. 17.2 Acute right
pontine ischaemic lesion on
diffusion weighted imaging

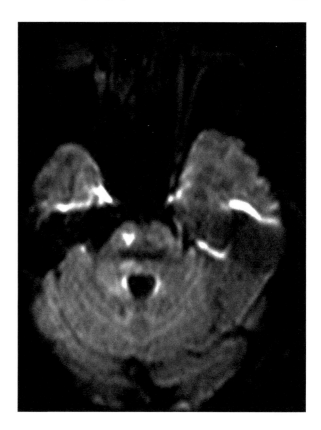

The patient was admitted to the Stroke Unit. The dose of aspirin was increased to 300 mg once daily. His speech recovered completely within 6 hours. The patient was concerned that the right carotid narrowing was the cause of the most recent event and needed early treatment. He was therefore referred to the vascular surgery team for review. No surgical operation was performed. It was concluded that his symptoms were secondary to the basilar artery stenosis and that the latter should be managed with intensive control of his vascular risk factors. He was discharged on the 4th day post admission on optimised secondary prevention treatment and with urgent follow up arranged with his stroke team in Italy.

Discussion

In patients with recent TIA or minor stroke secondary to ipsilateral internal carotid artery carotid stenosis greater than 50%, carotid endarterectomy reduced the risk of recurrent stroke secondary to significant stenosis by 17% in trials performed more than 20 years ago [1]. Surgery should be done as soon as possible after the symptomatic event, so long as the patient is neurologically and medically stable, and certainly where possible within 2 weeks of the presenting event. The evidence favouring from trials of carotid surgery for asymptomatic carotid stenosis is less convincing (4.1% gain over 5 years, 4.6% gain over 10 years) [2]. Medical therapy has improved considerably since these trials were done and there is ongoing recruitment to new international trials such as the Second European Carotid Surgery Trial (ECST-2) and the Asymptomatic Carotid Surgery Trial 2 (ACST2) to better understand the benefits of modern medical treatment compared with surgery in patients with carotid stenosis.

Many services cannot provide MRI as the initial imaging modality and busy stroke units under pressure to create beds for new admissions may consider that CT/CTA and carotid Doppler imaging, especially when concordant, are sufficient to make a diagnosis of symptomatic carotid stenosis even in the absence of an acute infarct on the admission CT. However, this may lead to misdiagnosis, as occurred in Italy in this case.

TIA by definition resolves within 24 hours and most last less than one hour. As a consequence, patients with TIA usually present to stroke services after the clinical deficit has resolved. This absence of objective abnormality at the time of first examination can lead to error in classification of the event as not being vascular in origin; or if TIA is thought likely, there may be mis-classification in terms of involved territory or mechanism of symptoms.

In this case, the examination on admission revealed only a mild dysarthria which is not itself diagnostic of a vascular cause and is not helpful in identifying the likely vascular territory of the symptoms [3]. The history of arm and leg involvement without associated involvement of the ipsilateral hemi-face most typically suggests a hemisphere capsular lacunar syndrome but perforator territory infarction in the pontine tegmentum causes identical deficits.

In this case the MRI demonstrated the site of the acute vascular lesion, which was not seen on CT. However MRI is not very sensitive for acute ischaemia lasting hours only [4] and restricted diffusion secondary to a TIA or minor stroke can reverse within days and might be missed by delayed MRI [5]. The admission CT showed background small vessel disease but no acute lesion but as it was performed at five hours post onset of the event, this might have been done before a small region of acute infarction in the basal ganglia or brainstem would be visible. In cases where MRI is not available or contraindicated, a delayed CT after 48 hours can sometimes be helpful in revealing acute infarction not seen on an early scan.

In this case, without MRI it is quite likely that the persuasive history of recurrent left hemiparesis in the context of an ulcerated stenosed right carotid stenosis would have led to carotid endarterectomy for an asymptomatic carotid stenosis.

Key Clinical Learning Points
1. Anatomical localisation of TIA or resolving ischaemic events can be difficult and benefits from a full and timely investigation, including MRI
2. Lacunar syndromes can be caused by ischaemia (or small haemorrhages) in the anterior or posterior circulation arterial territories
3. Patients with multiple vascular risk factors can exhibit multiple possible mechanisms for their stroke presentation. (In this case significant large and small vessel disease was identified on investigation)

Key Radiological Learning Points
1. CT scans performed very early into the course of a stroke presentation are most useful for identifying haemorrhage, alternative diagnoses and background pathology and less useful for identifying small new infarcts
2. Large artery disease can be present at multiple sites and the entire cerebrovascular anatomy should be imaged before decisions can be made about the relative importance of any one identified lesion
3. MRI is not very sensitive for demonstrating ischaemia in short lasting TIA and becomes less sensitive with time since event termination

References

1. Guay J, Ochroch EA. Carotid endarterectomy plus medical therapy or medical therapy alone for carotid artery stenosis in symptomatic or asymptomatic patients: a meta-analysis. J Cardiothorac Vasc Anesth. 2012;26(5):835–44. doi:10.1053/j.jvca.2012.01.044. Epub 2012 Apr 10.
2. Halliday A, Harrison M, Hayter E, et al. Asymptomatic Carotid Surgery Trial (ACST) Collaborative Group. 10-year stroke prevention after successful carotid endarterectomy for asymptomatic stenosis (ACST-1): a multicentre randomised trial. Lancet. 2010;376(9746): 1074–84. doi:10.1016/S0140-6736(10)61197-X.
3. Amort M, Fluri F, Schäfer J, et al. Transient ischemic attack versus transient ischemic attack mimics: frequency, clinical characteristics and outcome. Cerebrovasc Dis. 2011;32(1):57–64. doi:10.1159/000327034. Epub 2011 May 25.
4. Carpentier N, Edjlali M, Bouhafs F, et al. Serial brain MRI in TIA patients. J Neuroradiol. 2012;39(3):137–41. doi:10.1016/j.neurad.2012.02.002. Epub 2012 Jun 27.
5. Albach FN, Brunecker P, Usnich T, et al. Complete early reversal of diffusion-weighted imaging hyperintensities after ischemic stroke is mainly limited to small embolic lesions. Stroke. 2013;44(4):1043–8. doi:10.1161/STROKEAHA.111.676346. Epub 2013 Feb 28.

Chapter 18
Confusion After the 'Flu'

David Collas

Clinical History

A 46-year-old male teacher presented to his local Accident and Emergency department with a history of 3 days of drowsiness and confusion. He had been well until 7 weeks earlier, when he had a febrile illness attributed to influenza. He was slow to recover from this and continued to suffer from daily headaches of increasing frequency and severity. He also complained of persistent fatigue. His GP prescribed antibiotics for a presumed ear infection. His parents, with whom he was living, also reported transient episodes of disturbance of speech consisting of slurred speech, as well as "talking gibberish and texting nonsense". On one occasion, he failured to recognise them.

He had a history of type 1 diabetes mellitus diagnosed at the age of 22, complicated by diabetic retinopathy causing blindness in the right eye with reduced vision on the left. He had a 20 pack-year history of smoking cigarettes. There was no history of foreign travel, recent sexual exposure or use of recreational drugs.

Examination

On examination he was afebrile with a temperature of 35.5 °C. Systemic examination was normal. He was drowsy (Glasgow Coma Scale 14/15) and confused with a Mini-mental Test Score of 6/10. He had a left facial droop, slurred speech and left sided homonymous hemianopia. Power was symmetrical but limited by poor effort. Sensation was intact and the tendon reflexes were hard to elicit. The right plantar response was extensor.

D. Collas, BSc, MB, BS FRCP
Stroke Medicine, Watford General Hospital, Watford, UK
e-mail: david.collas@whht.nhs.uk

© Springer-Verlag London 2015

115

S.K. Gill et al. (eds.), *Stroke Medicine: Case Studies from Queen Square*,
DOI 10.1007/978-1-4471-6705-1_18

Within two days of admission he became disorientated in time, though remained orientated in place and person. He showed signs of an encephalopathy with slow processing, perseveration, poor organisation of thoughts and reduced awareness of surroundings; for instance he attempted to get back into a wet bed. He required constant prompting to attend to tasks and cooperate with assessment. He was able to follow one-stage commands and perform simple arithmetic and MMSE fell to 16/30. He became generally weak, more so on the left than the right, and was unable to lift either leg off the bed.

Investigations

On admission, FBC was normal but ESR was raised at 25 mm/h, as was CRP at 10.8 mg/l, (rising to 26.4 five days later). Liver enzymes were raised with alkaline phosphatase 206 U/l, gamma GT 159 IU/l, albumin 41 g/l. His renal function was impaired with urea 12.2 mmol/l, and creatinine 107 umol/l. He was hyperglycaemic with a blood glucose of 38.6 mmol/l, although he was not acidotic.

CT brain showed an infarct in right internal capsule (Fig. 18.1). MR with DWI demonstrated acute infarction in the left hypothalamus, left parietal lobe, right peri-ventricular white matter and in the genu of right internal capsule (Fig. 18.2).

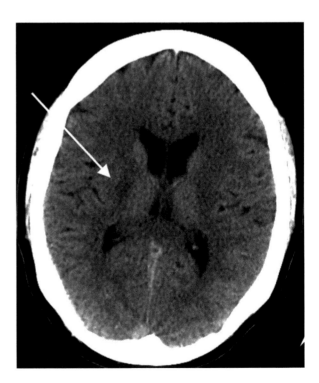

Fig. 18.1 CT on admission showing an acute infarct in the right internal capsule (*arrow*)

Fig. 18.2 FLAIR MRI showing bilateral cingulate gyrus cortical infarction in the ACA territory (*arrow*) and a small right periventricular infarct

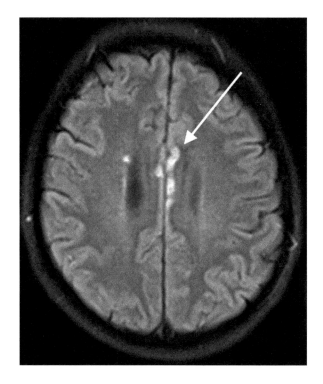

An EEG was reported as showing no seizure activity. CSF examination showed a raised opening pressure of 39 mmHg with a raised white cell count of 33 106/l (100% lymphocytes), and a raised protein of 0.76 g/l.

Clinical Progress

He became increasingly drowsy, with vacant episodes and was started on sodium valproate. On day 3 he was treated for possible herpes encephalitis in view of the preceding flu-like illness, progressive encephalopathy, and CSF findings, pending PCR and tests for vasculitis, which included ANA, ANCA, anti-DNA and anti-cardiolipin antibodies. These tests were all negative.

At this point diagnoses being considered include primary angiitis of the CNS, vascular cerebral lymphoma, and cerebral venous sinus thrombosis.

CT angiogram (Fig. 18.3) showed beading of intracranial arteries consistent with CNS vasculitis.

Unfortunately, he deteriorated rapidly and died before any further investigations could be performed.

A post-mortem examination was carried out. The findings on frozen sections were inconclusive and histology of fixated slices from the forebrain failed to yield

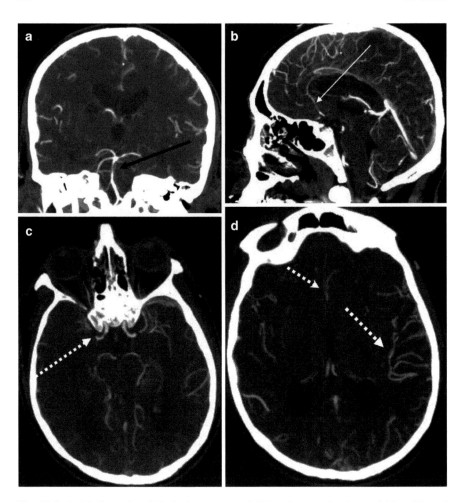

Fig. 18.3 Axial, Coronal and Sagittal sequences of CT angiogram showing variable calibre of small intracranial arteries involving (**a**) distal basilar artery (*black arrow*) (**b**) A2 segment (*solid white arrow*) (**c**) distal ICA (*dotted white arrow*) and (**d**) distal anterior and middle cerebral branches (*dashed white arrows*)

evidence of arteritis. However, when the posterior fossa was subsequently sectioned clear evidence of vasculitis was found with giant cells on microscopy. Examination of the temporal and other extra-cranial arteries confirmed that the vasculitis was confined to the intra-cerebral vessels. A final diagnosis of primary angiitis of the central nervous system was established.

Discussion

Primary angiitis of the CNS is a rare condition, with an incidence estimated at 1:2,000,000 [1–3]. It is twice as common in men as women, and is said to have an age of onset of over 40. The vasculitis is characterised by inflammation of small and medium sized arteries, leading to vessel occlusion and cerebral infarcts, but can cause haemorrhage, both intracerebral and subarachnoid. These cause focal symptoms in about 50% cases, which is preceded by headache in two thirds of cases, and often accompanied by encephalopathy. In the absence of treatment, the patient gradually declines with increasing encephalopathy and/or recurrent stroke. This conjunction of symptoms mimics many other CNS diseases.

MRI and CSF examination are essential initial investigations. High resolution MRI with contrast may reveal evidence of inflammation in the vessel walls, but the specificity of this finding remains to be confirmed [4]. Once other causes for similar presentations, including systemic vasculitis, have been ruled out, angiography and biopsy are required to confirm the diagnosis. Given the limitations in resolution of CTA this may require full conventional contrast angiography, which may show characteristic beading or multifocal narrowing of the larger arteries, which was well demonstrated in this case. However, this angiographic appearance is seen in other conditions including reversible vasoconstriction syndrome (see case 34), while angiography can be normal in proven vasculitis, especially if the pathology is confined to small vessels. Thus, it is our view that all patients with a strong suspicion of primary CNS angiitis should have a brain biopsy to establish the diagnosis prior to starting specific treatment because of the potential side effects of immunosuppression. However, given the patchy nature of the brain involvement even a biopsy may be negative. In positive cases, histology characteristically shows involvement of the leptomeninges and of veins and venules, all affected by mononuclear cell infiltration.

Secondary cerebral vasculitis can occur after viral infections such as Cytomegalavirus, Mycoplasma or Herpes zoster, and CSF should therefore be cultured for these organisms. CNS vasculitis has also been associated with Hepatitis B and HIV infection. Raised white cell count and protein are almost universal (90% cases). CNS vasculitis has been found in association with lymphoma and cerebral amyloid angiopathy, which may complicate interpretation of the histology.

Treatment is based on immunosuppression using steroids, and immunosuppressive agents, typically cyclophsophamide, which may have to be continued long term. It is helpful for neurologists and stroke physicians to discuss the management with a rheumatologist more used to treating vasculitis. With such treatment, long-term remission with successful withdrawal of treatment after 1 year has been reported.

Key Clinical Learning Points
1. Primary angiitis of the CNS typically has an insidious course with both focal and generalised clinical symptoms and signs
2. A history of gradual decline and chronic headache preceding cerebral infarction should prompt consideration of CNS vasculitis
3. Diagnosis of primary CNS angiitis can be impossible to confirm in life, even with a brain biopsy, due to patchy nature of the pathology
4. Blood tests can be entirely normal in CNS vasculitis if the disease is confined to the brain, and if biopsies are normal, it may be a diagnosis of exclusion

Key Radiological Learning Points
1. Brain MR is a necessary investigation and may show multifocal patchy infarction or haemorrhage and often shows involvement of deep white matter
2. Catheter angiography may be required to demonstrate the characteristic beading and irregularity of cerebral vessels seen in vasculitis, but may still be normal
3. True beading of intracranial vessels has to be distinguished from artefacts such as partial volume effect and other disorders such as reversible vasoconstriction syndrome
4. Contrast enhanced high resolution MRI can show enhancement of the walls of the large intracranial vessels, but the specificity of this finding remains to be established

References

1. Cravioto G, Feigin I. Noninfectious granulomatous angiitis with a predilection for the nervous system. Neurology. 1959;9:599–609.
2. Moore PM. The vasculitides. Curr Opin Neurol. 1999;12:383–8.
3. Caplan L, Louis D. Case histories of the Massachusetts general hospital case 10. N Engl J Med. 2000;342:957–65.
4. Küker W, Gaertner S, Nägele T, et al. Vessel wall contrast enhancement: a diagnostic sign of cerebral vasculitis. Cerebrovasc Dis. 2008;26:23–9.

Chapter 19
One Night with Venus, a Lifetime with Mars

Jeremy C.S. Johnson and Nicholas Losseff

Clinical History

A left-handed, 44-year-old retired city trader presented to the emergency department with a 2-day history of sudden onset of left hand and leg weakness. The weakness had been gradually worsening and he had sustained two falls. He described a 3-month prodrome of intermittent, severe right occipital headache that had been diagnosed as cluster headache. NSAIDs had proved ineffective, but there had been a good response to a 6-day course of high dose prednisolone.

He had also been seen in the rheumatology clinic 6 months previously with mild, intermittent pain affecting the distal joints of both hands. There had also been a pruritic rash affecting his chest and back. Rheumatological tests at the time including rheumatoid factor, anti-CCP antibodies and antinuclear antigen were negative. There were no vascular risk factors and his only other past medical history was of depression. He had no known drug allergies and had been taking prednisolone, ibuprofen and mirtazapine.

Examination

He was alert and orientated. Neurological examination revealed left facial weakness, with predominantly distal left arm weakness in a pyramidal distribution and mild weakness at the knee only in the lower limb. The reflexes were brisk bilaterally and the plantar responses were both equivocal. There was decreased sensation to

J.C.S. Johnson, MBBS, BSc • N. Losseff, MD, FRCP (✉)
Department of Stroke, National Hospital for
Neurology and Neurosurgery, London, UK
e-mail: nicholas.losseff@nhs.net

© Springer-Verlag London 2015
S.K. Gill et al. (eds.), *Stroke Medicine: Case Studies from Queen Square*,
DOI 10.1007/978-1-4471-6705-1_19

light touch in both his arm and leg, with sensory extinction in a similar distribution. His gait was mildly hemiparetic. Systems examination was unremarkable.

His observations were as follows – temperature 36.2, pulse 91, BP 144/99 mmHg, respiratory rate 16/min, and SpO$_2$ 96% on room air.

Investigations

Routine blood tests including fasting lipid profile were all within the normal range; his CRP was 4.6 mg/l., capillary blood glucose 5.3 mmol/l. An ECG showed sinus rhythm and his chest x-ray was normal.

CT (Fig. 19.1) showed a large heterogeneous lesion in the right frontal lobe, with an enhancing component anteriorly and surrounding hypoattenuation, which was likely to represent perilesional oedema. Within this there appeared to be a few streaky densities on the unenhanced scan which were thought to represent intralesional haemorrhage. The radiological impression was of a right frontal space-occupying lesion.

MRI (Fig. 19.2) showed a large area of restricted diffusion in the right middle cerebral artery territory involving the cortex, which was consistent with an MCA territory infarct. The T2* weighted sequence showed marked susceptibility artifact in the distal right M1 segment and M2 branches in the Sylvian fissure suggestive of

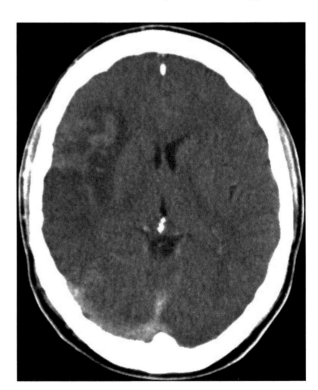

Fig. 19.1 Axial CT image post contrast showing large area of low density in right MCA territory with sparing of basal ganglia. There is pial/leptomeningeal enhancement at the margins of the lesion

Fig. 19.2 Axial T2 weighted image showing extensive area of signal change in right MCA territory involving grey and white matter

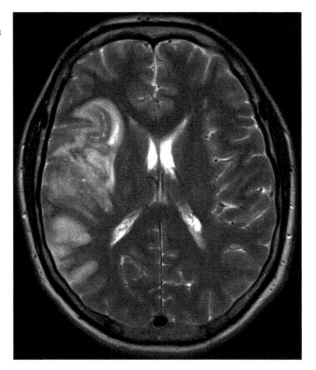

intravascular thrombus. There were, however, some unusual features associated with the infarct: in addition to the gyriform enhancement in the right frontal lobe and insula, there was also marked leptomeningeal enhancement in the Sylvian fissure and, to a lesser degree over the cerebral convexity. There was also some associated vasogenic oedema around the anterior aspect of the infarct, considered unusual and raising the possibility of an underlying inflammatory process, possibly infective or vasculitic.

A series of laboratory tests were as follows. Serum Treponema pallidum particle agglutination assay (TPPA) was positive at >1:1,280, Treponemal antibody enzyme immunoassay (EIA) and chemiluminescent microplate immunoassay (CMIA) were positive; serum Rapid Plasma Reagin (RPP) was positive at a titre of 1:16.

Tests for hepatitis B and C viruses, HIV, Toxoplasma, Herpes viruses, Varicella Zoster, Cytomegalovirus, Epstein-Barr virus and a Quantiferon Gold Test for tuberculosis were all negative. Serum ANA, ANCA and ACE were also negative. The syphilis serology was repeated with identical results.

A lumbar puncture was performed. CSF was clear and colourless; protein was 2.37 g/L and glucose 3.2 mmol/L. Both CSF and paired serum oligoclonal bands were positive. CSF RPR was negative, but TPPA was positive to a dilution of >1:1,280 and Treponemal antibody EIA was positive.

CSF cytology showed a large number of mature lymphocytes and occasional plasma cells, consistent with an inflammatory exudate; the findings were reported as consistent with chronic syphilitic infection with meningeal involvement.

CSF tests for Enteroviruses, Herpes 1 and 2, Varicella Zoster, Cytomegaloviurs, Epstein-Barr virus, Toxoplasma, microscopy for acid fast bacilli and polymerase chain reaction (PCR) for tubercle bacilli were all negative.

Based on clinical, radiological and laboratory findings, a diagnosis of meningovascular neurosyphilis was made.

Discussion

Despite a recent resurgence in the incidence of syphilis, it still remains a rare disease. 'Neurosyphilis' is an imprecise term used to indicate any syphilitic presence in the CNS that can range from asymptomatic patients with suggestive laboratory tests to 'classic' clinical syndromes that can be made at the bedside. As with all rare syndromes, it is highly prone to recruitment bias and the majority of published literature pertains to small case series that are often incomplete.

Giving meaningful prevalence estimates for meningovascular syphilis in the post penicillin era is therefore challenging, particularly as the interpretation of diagnostic tests becomes increasingly complex and nuanced as latency from index infection lengthens. To illustrate these points, in one retrospective cohort study of 3,270 patients with TIA or stroke, 4% had positive syphilis serology; of these however, only one patient was diagnosed with "definite" meningovascular syphilis, two with "probable" meningovascular syphilis and 34 "with positive serology without confirmation of neurosyphilis" [1].

The general rubric of neurosyphilis includes all pathological subdivisions of CNS involvement. This includes asymptomatic CNS involvement (positive serum tests with CSF pleocytosis), syphilitic meningitis, meningovascular syphilis, parenchymatous neurosyphilis (tabes dorsalis and general paresis) and gummatous neurosyphilis. It is useful to think of neurosyphilis as being predominantly meningeal, vascular or parenchymatous, depending on the clinical features present [2]. Syphilitic meningitis and meningovascular syphilis are both neuroinflammatory syndromes and show a degree of overlap. The former classically presents with signs of meningeal inflammation and patients may develop cranial nerve palsies and obstructive hydrocephalous; the latter is characterised by chronic meningitis and multifocal arteritis, with headache, apathy, irritability and focal neurological deficit reflecting the arterial territory involved.

Arteritis in meningovascular syphilis can affect large, medium or small arteries and arterioles. Histologically there is lymphocyte and plasma cell infiltration of the adventitia and media, with concentric, collagenous thickening of the intima causing stenosis and eventually occlusion or thrombus formation secondary to endothelial damage [3]. The middle cerebral artery tree is most commonly affected, often with large vessel infarction, but any of the intracranial vessels can be involved [4].

The often innocuous nature of primary infection with the spirochete Treponema pallidum, is hallmarked by an ulcerated painless chancre. The organism insinuates itself throughout the body and penetrates the CNS within hours of infection. Preferential multiplication occurs at the site of entry with localised lymphadenopathy that is usually painless; approximately 30% of patients having intercourse with infected partners will develop syphilis within 10–90 days.

The bacteraemic secondary phase is dominated by non-specific symptoms that may include headache, fever, sore throat, arthralgia and anorexia. In the skin, mucous patches, condylomata and a generalised rash of diverse manifestations are most characteristic. In both primary and secondary phases, symptoms typically resolve spontaneously within 1–6 weeks, but may recur in secondary syphilis. Tertiary syphilis develops in approximately one third of untreated patients and is characterised by organ specific involvement including heart, skin, bone and the CNS; this may occur anywhere from 5 to 20 years after the index infection.

The diagnosis of neurosyphilis is challenging and requires caution; laboratory tests are on the whole polarised as sensitive and non-specific, or the reverse. Direct visualisation of treponemes using dark field microscopy provides definitive evidence of syphilis infection if other pathogenic treponemes can be excluded (e.g. yaws and pinta) and remains the gold standard diagnostic laboratory test; large numbers of treponemes can be found at sites of local invasion, however, once disseminated this technique becomes impractical and insensitive.

Derivative tests are classified as treponemal or non-treponemal; treponemal antibody tests as a group have sensitivities approaching 100% (i.e. a negative test excludes neurosyphilis) and include Treponemal antibody EIA, TPPA, Treponema pallidum hemagglutination assay (TPHA), Fluorescent treponemal antibody absorption (FTA), microhemagglutination assay (MHA-TP) and more [5–7]. If neurosyphilis is a likely diagnosis, testing is recommended with treponemal tests first due to their high sensitivity, followed by more specific non-treponemal tests if the result is positive. All tests should include serum and CSF where possible.

Of the non-treponemal tests, the CSF Venereal Disease Research Laboratory (VDRL) test is probably the most widely used; it is highly specific, but insensitive, with false negative rates quoted as high as 50% [6, 7]. A recent study suggests the CSF-RPR test is as sensitive and specific as CSF VDRL [8]; CSF-RPR is currently used by the Public Health England reference laboratory in London.

A positive CSF VDRL is considered 'definitive' for neurosyphilis due to its high specificity, however its lack of sensitivity means it cannot be used to exclude the diagnosis if the pretest probability of neurosyphilis is considered moderate to high. The Centre for Disease Control and Prevention (CDC) takes this into account and defines 'definite' neurosyphilis as (1) any syphilis stage and (2) a reactive CSF-VDRL; presumptive neurosyphilis is defined as (1) any syphilis stage, (2) non-reactive CSF-VDRL, (3) elevated CSF protein or white blood cell count in the absence of other known abnormalities to cause this and (4) clinical symptoms or signs consistent with neurosyphilis in the absence of another likely diagnosis.

There is no single diagnostic imaging modality for neurosyphilis; imaging studies looking at CT and MRI findings in neurosyphilis are limited to small case series and demonstrate a multitude of findings. Meningovascular neurosyphilis has no characteristic features, with cortical and subcortical lesions, leptomeningeal enhancement, meningitis and arteritis all demonstrated. In a small recent case series using CT and MRI, 43% of patients with meningovascular syphilis had radiological evidence of stroke, both cortically and sub cortically in either the anterior or posterior circulations [9]. When intracranial arteritis is demonstrated, the middle cerebral artery is most commonly involved, followed by branches of the basilar artery [4, 9].

Penicillin remains the recommended treatment for all stages of syphilis; 3–4 million units of intravenous penicillin G, 4 hourly for 10–14 days, or 2.4 million units of procaine penicillin plus 50 mg of oral probenicid, four times a day for 10–14 days [6]. In penicillin allergic patients, ceftriaxone is a reasonable alternative [8].

The protean manifestations of syphilis is reflected in its historical moniker "the great imitator". Diagnosis is based on a combination of clinical, laboratory and imaging findings. Treponemal tests are highly sensitive, with poor specificity; they generally remain positive lifelong and do not distinguish syphilis from other treponemes. CSF testing with non-treponemal tests (VDRL, RPR) should only be pursued in the presence of reactive treponemal tests (TPPA, Treponemal antibody etc.). The wide error margin inherent in commonly used laboratory tests for syphilis is partly responsible for the uncertainty of epidemiological estimates for syphilis. Imaging findings are non-specific and may involve any vascular territory in meningovascular syphilis, with the MCA most commonly involved. It must be remembered that laboratory tests and imaging findings should support or refute a diagnosis, rather than make one. For the post penicillin generation, this is a timely reminder that syphilis still stalks the shadows and recesses of medicine, with characteristic subterfuge.

Key Clinical Learning Points
1. The re-emergence of syphilis warrants serious consideration in the differential diagnosis of atypical stroke, particularly in populations considered at risk
2. Neurosyphilis can present in myriad ways depending on the extent of meningeal and vascular involvement
3. Meningovascular syphilis is most commonly associated with stroke and is characterised by a large vessel arteritis typically affecting the middle cerebral artery
4. A negative treponemal test excludes syphilis and therefore testing should begin with a treponemal test, followed a non-treponemal test if positive
5. Treatment is with penicillin or ceftriaxone if penicillin allergic

Key Radiological Learning Points
1. Meningovascular syphilis has no characteristic features on CT and MRI
2. Cortical and subcortical infarction, leptomeningeal enhancement, meningitis and arteritis are all documented
3. Radiologically the most frequently involved artery is the middle cerebral artery followed by the basilar artery and it's branches

References

1. Cordato DJ, Djekic S, Taneja SR, et al. Prevalence of positive syphilis serology and meningo-vascular neurosyphilis in patients admitted with stroke and TIA from a culturally diverse population (2005–09). J Clin Neurosci. 2013;20(7):943–7. Epub 2013/05/15.
2. Branche GC. Diagnosis and treatment of neurosyphilis. J Natl Med Assoc. 1939;31(1):11–6. Epub 1939/01/01.
3. Ellison DL S, Chimelli L, Harding BA, et al. Neuropathology: a reference text of CNS pathology. 3rd ed. Elsevier; Oxford. 2013. 879 p.
4. Gallego J, Soriano G, Zubieta JL, et al. Magnetic resonance angiography in meningovascular syphilis. Neuroradiology. 1994;36(3):208–9. Epub 1994/04/01.
5. Harding AS, Ghanem KG. The performance of cerebrospinal fluid treponemal-specific antibody tests in neurosyphilis: a systematic review. Sex Transm Dis. 2012;39(4):291–7. Epub 2012/03/17.
6. Luger A, Schmidt BL, Steyrer K, et al. Diagnosis of neurosyphilis by examination of the cerebrospinal fluid. Br J Vener Dis. 1981;57(4):232–7. Epub 1981/08/01.
7. Larsen SA, Steiner BM, Rudolph AH. Laboratory diagnosis and interpretation of tests for syphilis. Clin Microbiol Rev. 1995;8(1):1–21. Epub 1995/01/01.
8. Marra CM. Update on neurosyphilis. Curr Infect Dis Rep. 2009;11(2):127–34. Epub 2009/02/26.
9. Peng F, Hu X, Zhong X, et al. CT and MR findings in HIV-negative neurosyphilis. Eur J Radiol. 2008;66(1):1–6. Epub 2007/07/14.

Chapter 20
A Hypertensive Spike

Asaipillai Asokanathan and Sumanjit K. Gill

Clinical History

A 30-year-old, right-handed man who worked as a builder was admitted with 3-day history of slurred speech, right facial droop and right arm incoordination and sensory loss. All of these symptoms had developed suddenly and did not progress. He described being unable to hold a cup properly and dropped it on two occasions, which was what prompted him to seek medical advice. There was no history of headache, neck pain or visual problems.

There was no significant past medical history, except hypertension diagnosed many years previously. However, he had never been started on antihypertensive medication. He was not on any prescribed medication or over the counter medication. There was no family history of stroke. He consumed 20 units of alcohol per week and admitted to taking 1–2 g of crack cocaine per week. Further questioning revealed that his last use of cocaine was 18 hours prior to the onset of symptoms when he had taken one gram of cocaine with alcohol.

Examination

He was alert and oriented. His blood pressure on admission was 205/112 mmHg with a regular pulse rate of 74/min. Heart sounds were normal. On neurological examination, he had right-sided facial weakness with pronator drift and finger-nose

A. Asokanathan, MRCP(UK), DGM(London)
Department of Stroke, East and North Hertfordshire NHS Trust, Stevenage, UK

S.K. Gill, BSc Hons, MBBS, MRCP (✉)
Education Unit, National Hospital for Neurology and Neurosurgery,
UCL Institute of Neurology, London, UK
e-mail: sumanjit.gill@nhs.net

© Springer-Verlag London 2015
S.K. Gill et al. (eds.), *Stroke Medicine: Case Studies from Queen Square*,
DOI 10.1007/978-1-4471-6705-1_20

ataxia of the right arm. His speech was intelligible and he had no language deficit. Fundus examination was normal. There was no nystagmus, dysdiadochokinesis or sensory deficit. His NIHSS on admission was 3.

Investigations

Routine blood investigations including a clotting screen were normal. His ESR was 10. ECG confirmed sinus rhythm, but there was no evidence of ischaemia or left ventricular hypertrophy. Chest X-ray was normal. CT showed a small deep haemorrhage in the left lentiform nucleus (Fig. 20.1). There was no evidence of underlying chronic hypertensive arteriopathy.

Intracranial and extracranial MRA were normal. Renal MRA showed a 'beading' appearance of the left renal artery suggestive of renal artery stenosis.

A diagnosis was made of left basal ganglia haemorrhage secondary to cocaine-induced acute hypertension. It remained uncertain whether he also had underlying chronic hypertensive arteriopathy secondary to renal artery stenosis.

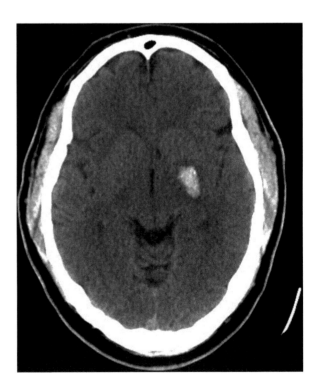

Fig. 20.1 Unenhanced CT showing acute haemorrhage in the left lentiform nucleus

Discussion

Cocaine is commonly taken via nasal insufflation and has a short half-life of around 60 min, which means that it is rapidly metabolised and not usually found on testing the urine. Its metabolites are however detectable for up to 14 days. Cocaine taken nasally reaches a peak concentration in the blood after 60 min, while crack cocaine reaches its peak level much more rapidly in 5–10 min. [1]

Cocaine use leads to an almost equal incidence of cerebral haemorrhage and ischaemic stroke. Both are more common with crack cocaine use and usually occur as an early complication within 24 hours of use. Cases of ICH and SAH have been known to occur within minutes to within the first hour after crack cocaine use. It should be recognised that cocaine commonly precipitates cerebral haemorrhage from an underlying vascular malformation, cerebral aneurysm or from chronic hypertensive vasculopathy. It is therefore essential to perform vascular imaging to exclude an underlying vascular lesion in patients with cocaine-induced stroke. The most likely mechanism for haemorrhagic stroke is an acute rise in blood pressure ('hypertensive spike') causing the rupture of underlying pathological lesion. In patients with no evident pathology on angiography, it is likely that the hypertensive spike induced by cocaine is sufficient to rupture a normal artery. Some studies have shown that there is a temporal relation with the type of stroke that will be suffered, in that shorter lead times to event are associated with ICH possibly because of extreme spikes in blood pressure [2].

The possible mechanisms for ischaemic stroke are multiple: cerebral artery vaso-constriction, cardiac arrhythmia, hypertensive spikes, enhanced platelet aggregation and in the long term with chronic use, accelerated atherosclerosis and cardiomyopa-thy [3]. In contrast to amphetamines it is almost never associated with vasculitis. Cocaine causes vasoconstriction by blocking the triple reuptake of serotonin-norepinephrine-dopamine. It has hydrophilic and lipophilic properties allowing it to cross the blood–brain barrier. A synergistic effect between cocaine and ethanol is also recognized, as in this case, because in the presence of ethanol, cocaine is metabolized to cocaethylene, which binds more powerfully to monoamine trans-porter proteins potentiating its effect [1].

In a series of 20 patients, ICH in those who had used cocaine was more fre-quently seen in the subcortical areas [4]. The most commonly affected areas are basal ganglia followed by thalamus, brainstem and cerebellum. One retrospective review of 45 patients found that cocaine related ICH was associated with increased mortality by 3 times in comparison to those with no history of cocaine use [5]. In an autopsy series of 26 patients with cocaine related ICH, 7 out of 19 cases did not have any evidence of chronic hypertensive arteriopathy in the brain [6]. This argues against a background of chronic hypertensive vasculopathy being the sole mecha-nism for ICH in this population. A more reasonable explanation could be due to a combination of cocaine related spikes in BP and a lowering of the upper limit of BP for cerebral autoregulation among cocaine users.

Key Clinical Learning Points
1. Cocaine use is associated with both ischaemic and haemorrhagic stroke – this usually occurs within 24 hours of ingestion
2. It is reasonable to screen for cocaine use in all young patients presenting with spontaneous ICH
3. Screening for secondary causes of hypertension should be undertaken in all patients

Key Radiological Learning Points
1. ICH in cocaine users is more commonly in sub cortical areas: most commonly affected are basal ganglia, thalamus, brainstem and cerebellum
2. Arterial vascular imaging is essential because 40% of cases are caused by hypertensive episodes combined with an underlying vascular lesions e.g. AVM or aneurysm

References

1. Treadwell SD, Robinson T. Cocaine use and stroke. Postgrad Med J. 2007;83(980):389–94.
2. Nanda A, Vannemreddy P, Willis B, et al. Stroke in the young: relationship of active cocaine use with stroke mechanism and outcome. Acta Neurochir Suppl. 2006;96:91–6.
3. Toosi S, Hess C, Hills NK, et al. Neurovascular complications of cocaine use in a tertiary stroke centre. J Stroke Cerebrovasc Dis. 2010;19(4):273–8.
4. Bajwa A, Silliman S, Crury J, et al. Characteristics and outcomes of cocaine-related spontaneous intracerebral haemorrhages. ISRN Neurology. 2013; vol. 2013, Article ID 124390, 5 pages. doi:10.1155/2013/124390.
5. Martin-Schild S, Albright KC, Hallevi H, et al. Intracerebral haemorrhage in cocaine users. Stroke. 2010;41:680–4.
6. Kibayashi K, Mastri AR, Hirsch CS. Cocaine induced intracerebral haemorrhage: analysis of predisposing factors and mechanisms causing haemorrhagic strokes. Hum Pathol. 1995;26(6): 659–63.

Chapter 21
Lying in Wait: Stroke and a Blistering Rash

Áine Merwick, Lucy Blair, Lionel Ginsberg, and Robert Simister

Clinical History

A 31-year-old right-handed man presented with left hand and left forearm sensory loss and right sided headache. Over the preceding week, he had experienced a flickering 'chequerboard' appearance in both eyes, lasting 1–2 min. The visual disturbance was binocular and was characterised by discrete gaps in his vision. The disturbance was intermittent and on each occasion lasted a number of minutes and then resolved. As it resolved, he experienced a headache over the right side of the head. The disturbance occurred two or three times a day. Around the same time period, he also experienced separately an auditory experience in which he heard an echo of his voice that would be as real to him as if he had repeated the sentence. This did not occur when others spoke to him.

Seven months previously he had an episode of shingles, diagnosed as ophthalmic herpes zoster, in the first division of the right trigeminal nerve, which had been treated with steroids and aciclovir. The symptoms at the time were characterised by severe pain around and behind the right eye, with a blistering rash over the right

Á. Merwick, MB, BMed Sc, MSc, PhD, MRCPI
Department of Neurology, National Hospital for Neurology
and Neurosurgery, Queen Square, London, UK
e-mail: aine.merwick@uclh.nhs.uk

L. Blair, MBChB, BMedSci
Hyper Acute Stroke Unit, University College Hospital, London, London, UK

L. Ginsberg, BSc, MB BS, PhD, FRCP, FHEA
Department of Neurology, Royal Free Hospital, London, UK

R. Simister, MA, FRCP, PhD (✉)
Comprehensive Stroke Service, National Hospital for Neurology
and Neurosurgery, UCLH Trust, London, UK
e-mail: robert.simister@nhs.net

© Springer-Verlag London 2015
S.K. Gill et al. (eds.), *Stroke Medicine: Case Studies from Queen Square*,
DOI 10.1007/978-1-4471-6705-1_21

temple. He had some transient visual disturbance at time of the acute infection and subsequently developed a suspected secondary skin infection. He was started on aciclovir approximately two days after onset of these symptoms. He was referred to an ophthalmologist and was prescribed a sustained course of topical steroid eye drops and topical antiviral eye drops.

He had no family history of vascular disease and no previous history of thrombotic events, joint problems, smoking, recreational drug use or immunosuppressive illness. He had no history of hypertension, diabetes mellitus or hypercholesterolaemia.

Examination

On examination, his blood pressure was 161/100 mmHg and his temperature was 37.4 °C. His heart rate was regular at 97 beats per minute with normal heart sounds and no audible cardiac murmur. There were no skin lesions. The optic fundi were normal and eye movements were full, with no double vision. Visual fields were full to confrontation on bedside testing and the remainder of cranial nerve examination was normal. Power in the upper and lower limbs was normal. Deep tendon reflexes were symmetrical. The plantar responses were flexor. There were no sensory deficits. National Institute of Health Stroke Score (NIHSS) was 0. He scored 28/30 on the Montreal Cognitive Assessment (MoCA) questionnaire, losing points for delayed recall and attention, as well as having mildly reduced verbal fluency.

Investigations

CT showed an acute/subacute cortical infarct involving the right temporal lobe including the temporal operculum, with further smaller infarcts in the posterior right temporal lobe. CTA showed high-grade stenosis of the proximal right M1 branch of MCA and stenosis of the supraclinoid right ICA, but no intracranial occlusion. The aortic arch, subclavian arteries, and vertebral arteries were normal.

MRI showed multiple cortical infarcts within the right MCA territory, involving the temporal lobe, the parieto-occipital junction, and mature cortical damage within the right inferior parietal lobule with some haemosiderin deposition, in keeping with a mature MCA infarct, suggestive of a prior ischaemic event in the same vascular territory (Fig. 21.1) MRA showed flow attenuation and contrast enhancement in the supraclinoid right ICA extending into the proximal right M1 branch of MCA (Fig. 21.2).

His total cholesterol was 5.8 mmol/l, HDL 1.1 mmol/l, LDL 4.0 mmol/l, glucose 5.2 mmol/l, and ESR 8. Serological tests for thrombophilia, inflammatory markers, HIV, hepatitis B, hepatitis C and autoimmune profiles were negative. ECG showed sinus rhythm, and cardiac monitoring was also normal. Echocardiography was

Fig. 21.1 MRI axial DWI image shows multiple cortical infarcts within the right middle cerebral territory, involving the temporal lobe and the parieto-occipital junction

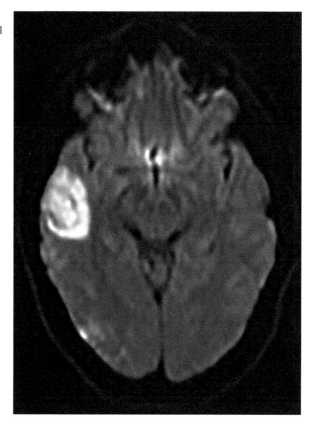

normal with good global systolic function and an estimated left ventricular ejection fraction of 69%.

CSF examination was normal with a protein concentration of 0.54 g/L. CSF varicella zoster virus (VZV) PCR and VZV IgG were negative. Serum examination for VZV IgG was positive, while serum VZV IgM was negative; suggestive of previous infection.

He was diagnosed as having VZV intracranial vasculopathy. He was treated acutely with intravenous aciclovir, followed by oral valciclovir to complete a 21 day course of anti-viral therapy, along with a tapering course of oral steroids starting at 90 mg/kg, reducing by 5 mg. He was also commenced on an antiplatelet agent (clopidogrel 75 mg) and a statin (atorvastatin 40 mg).

MRI and MRA 2 months later showed persistent right ICA wall thickening and signal change extending into the right MCA with vessel enhancement and flow attenuation. Positron emission tomography (PET) CT scan performed 3 months after the stroke presentation did not show any enhancement. No stroke recurrence occurred over a period of 18 months follow up and he made an excellent functional recovery.

Fig. 21.2 MRA shows attenuated flow signal in the supraclinoid right internal carotid artery and right middle cerebral artery

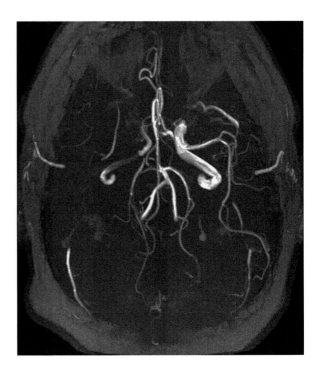

Discussion

Stroke following infection with varicella zoster virus (VZV) also known as herpes zoster, is a well-recognised complication of childhood chicken pox infection. The Greek word hérpēs, literally meaning 'to creep', describes the cutaneous lesions.

VZV vasculopathy can present as ischaemic or haemorrhagic stroke, aneurysm with and without haemorrhage, venous sinus thrombosis, or spinal cord infarction. [1, 2]. It is important to recognize that these variants can present without rash [3]. Vigilance for this potentially treatable vasculopathy is pivotal as it may occur up to several months after infection or re-activation [4, 5].

VZV is known to replicate in arteries. After the acute infection, the virus persists in a non-infectious latent form in ganglia along the neuraxis, with intermittent periods of reactivation. Both primary infection and secondary reactivation are associated with stroke [6].

Stroke related to zoster infection is less well recognised in adults, although epidemiological data suggests VZV increases stroke risk acutely by 127% in the first 2 weeks, and by 17% between 2 weeks and 1 year after viral symptoms, and that herpes zoster is an independent risk factor for vascular disease particularly for stroke, TIA, and MI in subjects affected by VZV before the age of 40 years [7, 8]. Herpes zoster ophthalmicus (HZO) in one study were found to have a 4.52-fold (95% confidence interval 2.45–8.33) higher risk of stroke than the matched comparison cohort, in a health insurance registry within a population-based dataset. In the same study, there was no significant difference in the rate of stroke development between patients who had received systemic antiviral treatment and those who had not [9]. A UK clinical practice research database study showed the stroke rate was increased following zoster compared with the baseline unexposed period, then gradually reduced over 6 months: with an age-adjusted incidence ratios of 1.63 (95% CI, 1.32–2.02) in weeks 1–4, 1.42 (95% CI 1.21–1.68) in weeks 5–12, and 1.23 (95% CI, 1.07–1.42) in weeks 13–26, with no increase thereafter [10]. A stronger effect was observed for individuals with zoster ophthalmicus, rising to a >3-fold rate 5–12 weeks after zoster. In one observational study oral antivirals were given to 55% of individuals: incidence ratios of stroke were lower among those receiving antivirals compared with those not treated, suggesting a potential protective effect [10].

As in our case, CSF pleocytosis is not required to diagnose VZV vasculopathy and only approximately 30% of cases have CSF VZV DNA detected. Specific intra-thecal synthesis of anti-VZV antibodies may be a useful marker of zoster infection. Detection of anti-VZV IgG antibodies in CSF has been reported in up to 93% of patients in one study of adult patients [4]. In paediatric studies, up to 100% of children with stroke attributed to primary chicken pox had detectable anti-VZV IgG antibodies in CSF [11].

In this case, other causes of vasculopathy were considered including inflammation, connective tissues diseases and other infections. Dissection or premature causes of atherosclerosis were also considered as a possible cause of large vessel vasculopathy. The preceding history of herpes zoster in the ipsilateral trigeminal nerve and carotid artery distribution was considered to be clinically relevant. The presence of infarcts of different ages suggested that there may have been ischaemic events around the time of the initial episode of herpes zoster ophthalmicus with subsequent ischaemia prompting the later hospital attendance.

Peri-infectious and post infectious vasculitis and vasculopathy has been reported in fungal, bacterial and spirochete as well as viral infections (specifically in Lyme disease, tuberculosis, syphilis, and histoplasmosis) [12–15]. An increased peri-infection stroke risk has been described in association with other systemic infections, and infection along with inflammation has been associated with increased atherosclerosis risk [12, 16]. Acute infection (odds ratio 5.1 [3.5–7.3]) has been identified as an independent risk predictor of stroke amongst TIA patients included in the Austrian Stroke registry [16]. A relationship between infection, vasculopathy and stroke in other viral infections including HIV and CMV has also been suggested [1, 12, 17]. Increased stroke risk in adult and paediatric patients with HIV has been reported, but it not clear whether HIV directly causes a vasculopathy or if the associated immunosuppression facilitates ongoing infections by organisms that are known to cause vasculopathy e.g. *Herpes zoster* or syphilis [1, 18–20]. In the setting of suspected VZV vasculopathy, testing for HIV or underlying immunosuppression might be prudent. Differentiating between VZV vasculopathy and co-existent HIV is challenging in practice, although one small case series has suggested deep-seated ischaemic infarcts are more frequently seen in VZV vasculopathy than in HIV vasculopathy amongst patients with HIV [17].

Both large and small arteries are commonly affected in VZV vasculopathy, followed in frequency by small arteries alone, and, least often, by large arteries alone [1]. More than one artery is usually involved, and thus may result in a multifocal vasculopathy with moyamoya-like features [21]. Vessel wall enhancement may be detected and typical angiographic changes include segmental constriction, often with post-stenotic dilatation. Deep infarcts are more common than superficial infarction and white matter more is commonly affected than grey matter. Temporal artery histology has shown inflammation and VZV DNA in multiple regions, and the presence of VZV antigen, has also been shown in temporal artery samples from some patients with clinical features suggestive of giant cell arteritis [22, 23].

Management of VZV vasculopathy is a challenge both diagnostically and therapeutically as the optimal duration of antiviral treatment and the role of steroids is unclear. Steroids in bacterial infections have been shown to reduce inflammation, which is a leading cause of disability associated with meningitis. In viral infections the role of steroids is less clear. Some authors have hypothesised that steroids may in fact prolong infection. However, histologic specimens often demonstrate an inflammatory response in infected cerebral arteries and oral prednisone (1 mg/kg daily for 5 days) without a steroid taper has been suggested by some experts [2]. The largest case series to date consisted of 30 patients who were treated with antiviral therapy, steroids, or both [4]. In those treated with aciclovir alone, 66% had neurological deficits that improved or stabilized, compared with 75% who improved or stabilized when treated with both aciclovir and steroids [4].

It is suggested immunocompetent patients with VZV vasculopathy should be treated with a full 14-day course of intravenous aciclovir, 10–15 mg/kg given three times daily [2]. Immunocompromised patients or those with recurrent VZV vasculopathy may need a longer course. Determination of the optimal dose, route, and duration of antiviral treatment, and benefit of concurrent steroid therapy awaits large prospective studies [2].

Based on the most recent epidemiological data available VZV vasculopathy may be a greater public health issue that previously appreciated and as a vaccine is now available, the primary infection is potentially preventable [10].

Key Clinical Learning Points
- Acute and subacute stroke risk is increased up to 5 fold following herpes zoster infection
- CSF features may include pleocytosis, intrathecally-produced VZV-specific IgG, or abnormal CSF PCR with detection of VZV DNA
- Treatment with intravenous aciclovir is recommended for 14 days
- In patients presenting with VZV vasculopathy underlying immunosuppression must be looked for
- Residual vessel abnormalities may persist or may be first detected months after the acute infection/reactivation

Key Radiological Learning Points
- VZV vasculopathy manifests as a large artery obliterative vasculopathy that can resemble moyamoya syndrome
- Vessel wall enhancement may be detected
- Typical angiographic changes include segmental constriction, often with post-stenotic dilatation
- Deep infarcts are more common than superficial infarction
- White matter is more commonly affected than grey matter
- The grey–white matter junctions are commonly affected
- VZV vasculopathy may present also with subarachnoid haemorrhage, cerebral haemorrhage or with carotid dissection

References

1. Nagel MA, Mahalingam R, Cohrs RJ, et al. Virus vasculopathy and stroke: an under-recognized cause and treatment target. Infect Disord Drug Targets. 2010;10(2):105–11.
2. Gilden D, Cohrs RJ, Mahalingam R, et al. Varicella zoster virus vasculopathies: diverse clinical manifestations, laboratory features, pathogenesis, and treatment. Lancet Neurol. 2009;8(8):731.
3. Russman AN, Lederman RJ, Calabrese LH, et al. Multifocal varicella zoster virus vasculopathy without rash. Arch Neurol. 2003;60:1607–9.
4. Nagel MA, Cohrs RJ, Mahalingam R, et al. The varicella zoster virus vasculopathies: clinical, CSF, imaging, and virologic features. Neurology. 2008;70(11):853–60.
5. Bodensteiner JB, Hille MR, Riggs JE. Clinical features of vascular thrombosis following varicella. Am J Dis Child. 1992;146(1):100–2.
6. Bartolini L, Gentilomo C, Sartori S, et al. Varicella and stroke in children: good outcome without steroids. Clin Appl Thromb Hemost. 2011;17(6):E127–30.
7. Sreenivasan N, Basit S, Wohlfahrt J, et al. The short- and long-term risk of stroke after herpes zoster – a nationwide population-based cohort study. PLoS One. 2013;8(7):e69156.
8. Breuer J, Pacou M, Gauthier A, et al. Herpes zoster as a risk factor for stroke and TIA. A retrospective cohort study in the UK. Neurology. 2014;82(3):206–12.
9. Lin HC, Chien CW, Ho JD. Herpes zoster ophthalmicus and the risk of stroke: a population-based follow-up study. Neurology. 2010;74:792–7.
10. Langan SM, Minassian C, Smeeth L, et al. Risk of stroke following herpes zoster: a self-controlled case-series study. Clin Infect Dis. 2014;58(11):1497–503.
11. Miravet E, Danchaivijitr N, Basu H, et al. Clinical and radiological features of childhood cerebral infarction following varicella zoster virus infection. Develop Med Child Neurol. 2007; 49(6):417–22.
12. Elkind MS. Inflammatory mechanisms of stroke. Stroke. 2010;41(10 Suppl):S3–8.
13. Lebas A, Toulgoat F, Saliou G, et al. Stroke due to lyme neuroborreliosis: changes in vessel wall contrast enhancement. J Neuroimaging. 2012;22(2):210–2.
14. Chahine LM, Khoriaty RN, Tomford WJ, et al. The changing face of neurosyphilis. Int J Stroke. 2011;6(2):136–43.
15. Nguyen FN, Kar JK, Zakaria A, et al. Isolated central nervous system histoplasmosis presenting with ischemic pontine stroke and meningitis in an immune-competent patient. JAMA Neurol. 2013;70(5):638–41.

16. Ferrari J, Knoflach M, Kiechl S, et al. Early clinical worsening in patients with TIA or minor stroke: the Austrian Stroke Unit Registry. Neurology. 2010;74:136–41.
17. Gutierrez J, Ortiz G. HIV/AIDS patients with HIV vasculopathy and VZV vasculitis: a case series. Clin Neuroradiol. 2011;21(3):145–51.
18. Patsalides AD, Wood LV, Atac GK, et al. Cerebrovascular disease in HIV-infected pediatric patients: neuroimaging findings. AJNR Am J Roentgenol. 2002;179(4):999–1003.
19. Schieffelin JS, Williams PL, Djokic D, et al. Central nervous system vasculopathy in HIV-infected children enrolled in the pediatric AIDS clinical trials group 219/219C study. J Pediatr Infect Dis. 2013;2(1):50–6.
20. Benjamin LA, Bryer A, Emsley HC, et al. HIV infection and stroke: current perspectives and future directions. Lancet Neurol. 2012;11(10):878–90.
21. Ueno M, Oka A, Koeda T, et al. Unilateral occlusion of the middle cerebral artery after varicella-zoster virus infection. Brain Dev. 2002;24(2):106–8.
22. Kleinschmidt-DeMasters BK, Gilden DH. Varicella-Zoster virus infections of the nervous system: clinical and pathologic correlates. Arch Pathol Lab Med. 2001;125(6):770.
23. Nagel MA, Bennett JL, Khmeleva N, et al. Multifocal VZV vasculopathy with temporal artery infection mimics giant cell arteritis. Neurology. 2013;80:2017–21.

Chapter 22
An Unusual Case of Paradoxical Embolus

Sumanjit K. Gill and Nicholas Losseff

Clinical History

A 62-year-old gentleman was electively admitted for laparoscopic robotic prostatectomy, to treat localised prostate carcinoma. He had no other past medical history. His pre-operative assessment was unremarkable and the only investigations performed were a routine set of blood tests, which were normal and a 12-lead ECG which showed him to be in sinus rhythm with left axis deviation but no hypertrophy. The surgery (during which he was in lithotomy in the Trendelenberg position i.e. lying supine with his feet 30° higher than the head) was uneventful. He was transferred back to the ward but around 8 hours later was noted to be still drowsy, a state originally ascribed to the general anaesthetic, which had been administered earlier.

Examination

He was drowsy but opened his eyes to pain. He was not vocalising. He had a gaze preference towards the right side. He had a left hemiparesis and neglect. There was an extensor plantar response on the left side, the right plantar response was flexor. His blood pressure was 150/70 mmHg and his pulse was regular.

S.K. Gill, BSc Hons, MBBS, MRCP (✉)
Education Unit, National Hospital for Neurology and Neurosurgery,
UCL Institute of Neurology, London, UK
e-mail: sumanjit.gill@nhs.net

N. Losseff, MD, FRCP
Department of Stroke, The National Hospital for Neurology and Neurosurgery, London, UK

Investigations and Clinical Progress

CT (Fig. 22.1) confirmed the clinical suspicion of a right MCA territory infarct. There was visible thrombus in the right middle cerebral artery but he was out of the time window for either thrombolysis or endovascular treatment, and of course had also just undergone major surgery. A subsequent MRI is shown in Fig. 22.2.

Further investigation for possible causes of his stroke included a 24 hours tape which showed occasional ventricular ectopics but no arrhythmia. MRA of the neck and intracranial vessels was normal. His fasting glucose was normal and total cholesterol 4.4 mmol/L. A bubble echocardiogram was strongly positive for a patent foramen ovale (PFO) on valsalva and there was a highly mobile intra-arterial septum.

He recovered rapidly despite radiological appearances of a large infarct. When discharged a week later he was independently mobile and his cognition was intact. There was some persisting upper limb weakness for which he continued to have physiotherapy in the community.

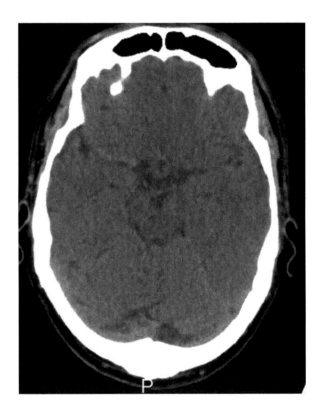

Fig. 22.1 Unenhanced CT scan – hyperdense clot is visible in the right middle cerebral artery

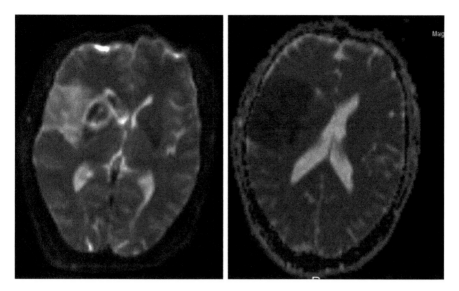

Fig. 22.2 Axial diffusion weighted imaging: B1000 DWI (*left*) and ADC map (*right*) show matched defect in the right middle cerebral artery territory indicating an acute infarct

Discussion

PFO is an overrepresented finding in patients who have had "cryptogenic" stroke (up to 50% [1]) and might be a risk factor for recurrent stroke [2]. However, the recurrence rate in patients treated with aspirin is very low, unless the PFO is associated with an atrial septal aneurysm [3]. In one cardiac autopsy study the overall incidence in the normal general population was 27.3% and decreased with age. The size of the PFO increased with age [4].

The most common causes of cryptogenic stroke are cardioembolic: paroxysmal atrial fibrillation (AF), valvular heart disease and septal defects. The detection of AF may require very prolonged monitoring. Mechanisms for stroke in those with PFO include paradoxical embolus from the deep veins, thrombus generated by cardiac arrhythmia or local formation of thrombus within the PFO, which is a tunnel rather an hole, between the atria. Paradoxical embolus is also associated with atrial septal defects, ventricular septal defects and pulmonary arteriovenous fistulae. Possible treatment strategies are that of closure (either open or percutaneous), antiplatelet therapy or anticoagulantion.

The value of closure is currently uncertain because recent randomised trials have shown that there is no definite reduction after percutaneous closure of the PFO in the risk of recurrent cerebrovascular events [5-7]. However, it is difficult to draw categorical conclusions from because of low event rates and there was heterogeneity within the treatment options across the groups studied.

In clinical practice, our practice is that each case is considered by a multidisciplinary team and decision-making is based upon considering all the other risk factors for stroke and the likely risk of recurrence. A scoring system which takes additional patient factors into account in order to aid clinical decision-making is the RoPE score [7]. Complications of the procedure need to be considered and the rate is anything up to 6%, these include: device embolus, pericardial effusion, air embolism. From the public health perspective the question remains not whether PFO is a risk factor or cause for stroke, but whether the benefits of treatment with closure outweigh the risks. Only careful and appropriately recruited clinical trials can answer this question and where such trials are open, the appropriate management is to randomise patients without bias.

It has been suggested in the past that PFO may also be associated with migraine and that closure may bring some relief to intractable migraine. In a meta analysis of 11 studies found that closure led to complete cure in 46% of patients and significant resolution in 83% [8]. Whilst it is likely that a PFO may trigger or cause migraine in some patients, the majority of patients with migraine have a genetic cause and co-incidental PFO.

Key Clinical Learning Points
1. PFO is associated with a risk of recurrent stroke particularly when associated with an atrial septal aneurysm
2. Strokes can arise from in situ thrombus formation, paradoxical embolus or by triggering atrial arrhythmias
3. Closure should be considered if it is implicated in the cause of stroke but may not be clearly beneficial so an alternative cause must be clearly ruled out
4. PFO is more common in those with migraines and closure may help relieve these as well as contributing to reducing stroke risk

---

Key Radiological Learning Points
1. Cardioembolic infarcts are usually large infarcts, they can affect multiple arterial territories and both hemispheres
2. A hyperdense middle cerebral artery can be the earliest sign of stroke. Drug thrombolysis is relatively ineffective in large artery thrombotic occlusion and the role of endovascular thrombectomy is emerging as a promising hyperacute treatment in this patient group

References

1. Homma S, Sacco RL. Patent foramen ovale and stroke. Circulation. 2005;112:1063–72.
2. Mas JL, Arquizan C, Lamy C, et al. Recurrent cerebrovascular events associated with PFO, atrial septal aneurysm or both. N Engl J Med. 2001;345:1740–6.
3. Hagen PT, Scholz DG, Edwards WD. Incidence and size of patent foramen ovale during the first ten decades of life: an autopsy study of 965 hearts. Mayo Clin Proc. 1984;59(1):17–20.
4. Furlan AJ, Reisman M, Massaro J, et al. Closure or medical therapy for cryptogenic stroke with patent foramen ovale. N Engl J Med. 2012;366:991–9.
5. Carroll JD, Saver JL, Thaler DE, et al. Closure of patent foramen ovale versus medical therapy after cryptogenic stroke. N Engl J Med. 2013;368:1092–100.
6. Meier B, Kalesan B, Mattle H, et al. Percutaneous closure of patent foramen ovale in cryptogenic embolism. N Engl J Med. 2013;368:1083–91.
7. Kent DM, Thaler DE, et al. The Risk of Paradoxical Embolus (RoPE) Study: developing risk models for application to ongoing randomised trials of percutaneous patent foramen ovale for cryptogenic stroke. Trials. 2011;12:185.
8. Butera G, Biondi Zoccai GGL, Carminati M, et al. Systematic review and meta analysis of currently available clinical evidence and migraine and patent foramen ovale percutaneous closure: much ado about nothing. Catheter Cardiovasc Interv. 2010;75(4):494–504.

Chapter 23
Reaching a Crescendo

Sumanjit K. Gill

Clinical History

A 69-year-old gentleman presented to the emergency department with acute left sided weakness. The first episode had occurred 2 hours earlier, when whilst he was seated he found he was unable to reach for his glasses. This resolved in under a minute but recurred 2 hours later. His wife called an ambulance and he had another episode whilst on the way to hospital. He had no past medical history other than being an occasional cigarette smoker.

Examination

On arrival he was alert and gave a good account of events. He had dysarthria and left facial weakness. Visual fields were intact. He had a dense left hemiparesis. There was no sensory deficit or inattention. His left plantar response was extensor. His cardiovascular examination was normal although his blood pressure was elevated at 170/80 mmHg. His admission CT was normal (Fig. 23.1) and he was treated with intravenous thrombolysis.

S.K. Gill, BSc Hons, MBBS, MRCP
Education Unit, National Hospital for Neurology and Neurosurgery,
UCL Institute of Neurology, London, UK
e-mail: sumanjit.gill@nhs.net

© Springer-Verlag London 2015
S.K. Gill et al. (eds.), *Stroke Medicine: Case Studies from Queen Square*,
DOI 10.1007/978-1-4471-6705-1_23

Fig. 23.1 Initial unenhanced
CT scan

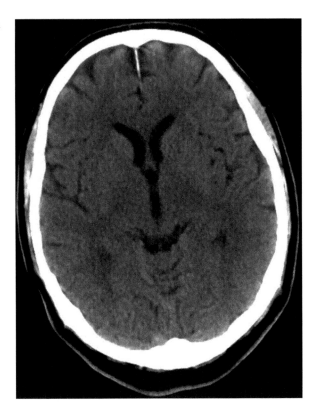

Investigations and Clinical Progress

He was reviewed 2 hours post treatment and his weakness had completely resolved. However, the night team were called to review him as his weakness recurred 12 hours later – it was complete and again affecting the left side. By the time a repeat scan is arranged the symptoms had resolved. In the morning he had yet another relapse of his symptoms – his CT scan is shown below (Fig. 23.2). This showed an evolving right hemisphere capsular infarct. He was given high dose dual antiplatelet therapy, but unfortunately this time his weakness persisted. His 24-hours post thrombolysis CT is shown below (Fig. 23.3) – the diagnosis of a capsular warning syndrome was confirmed. He progressed to a rehabilitation unit and on review at 2 weeks was independently mobile with only a minimal residual deficit.

Discussion

Capsular warning syndrome has a dramatic presentation consisting of crescendo TIAs and often (42% in one series [1]) culminating in an internal capsule or pontine infarct. It was first described in 1993 [1] in a patient who had recurrent subcortical

Fig. 23.2 CT head demonstrating a right hemisphere lacunar infarct

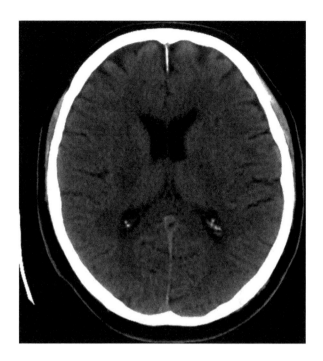

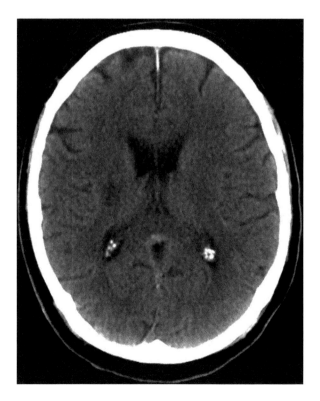

Fig. 23.3 CT scan at 24 hours post presentation – an established right hemisphere capsular infarct

events. The precise mechanism is not defined although it has been postulated that it may be due to haemodynamic changes resulting in underperfusion of an atheromatous or otherwise diseased lenticulostriate artery. Most lenticulostriate arteries arise from the middle cerebral artery and one case has been reported where angioplasty of a stenosed middle cerebral artery has restored flow to these arteries and terminated recurrent TIAs.

It has been found that capsular warning TIAs are usually refractory to medical treatment with either thrombolytics or heparin, although a report of 4 cases suggested that intravenous thrombolysis given during an attack might prevent progression to infarction in some patients [2]. Common practice in the UK is to give dual high dose antiplatelet therapy in order to stop the progression to an infarct, but as was seen in this case they can also be ineffective in this situation [3]. In view of the possible haemodynamic component, blood pressure should be maintained with the judicious use of intravenous fluids. In addition to the capsular warning syndrome, many lacunar syndromes, stutter or progress over several days. Again this progression is often refractory to optimal medical management.

Key Clinical Learning Points
1. Capsular warnings present with a stereotyped recurrent weakness and carry a high risk of completed stroke
2. During an event thrombolytic therapy might prevent the progression to a full stroke
3. Blood pressure should be maintained with intravenous fluids to ensure adequate cerebral perfusion. There is no role for pressor agents

Key Radiological Learning Points
1. The area of ischaemia is usually in the internal capsule but can also be pontine and an MRI may be more useful than CT in visualising the infarct after the stroke has completed

References

1. Donnan GA, O'Malley HM, Quang L, Hurley S, Bladin PF. The capsular warning syndrome: pathogenesis and clinical features. Neurology. 1993;43(5):957–62.
2. Vivanco-Hidalgo RM, Rodriguez-Campello A, Ois A, et al. Thrombolysis in capsular warning syndrome. Cerebrovasc Dis. 2008;25:508–10.
3. Fahey DC, Alberts MJ, Berstein RA. Oral clopidogrel load in aspirin-resistant capsular warning syndrome (abstract). Cerebrovasc Dis. 2004;17:8.

Chapter 24
Bihemispheric Infarcts

Rupert Oliver and Richard Perry

Clinical History

A 70-year-old Solicitor's Clerk was found lying in the street near a grocery store with his shopping bags strewn on the ground around him. He reported having dropped them from his left hand shortly before falling over but was unable to recall how long ago this happened and the fall was unwitnessed. He was found to be 'FAST' positive by the attending paramedics and was taken urgently to the nearest hyperacute stroke unit. He had a background history of hypertension and basal cell carcinoma but was otherwise well.

Examination

He was disoriented, with slurred speech and a mild left hemiparesis. He appeared cachectic but was afebrile and had a blood pressure of 164/84 mmHg.

R. Oliver, PhD, MRCP (✉)
Department of Neurology, Guy's and St. Thomas' Hospitals, St. Thomas' Hospital, London, UK
e-mail: rupert.oliver@gstt.nhs.uk

R. Perry, BM, BCh, MA, PhD, MRCP(UK)
Department of Neurology, National Hospital for Neurology & Neurosurgery, London, UK

© Springer-Verlag London 2015
S.K. Gill et al. (eds.), *Stroke Medicine: Case Studies from Queen Square*,
DOI 10.1007/978-1-4471-6705-1_24

151

Investigations and Clinical Progress

An ECG showed sinus rhythm. CT head with CT angiography of the head and neck revealed no abnormalities. His CRP was raised at 37 mg/l and his white cell count was markedly elevated at 24×10^9/l (a neutrophilia). He had an elevated ESR of 107 mm/hour; but a vasculitic screen (including ANA, ANCA, dsDNA and complement levels) was negative.

As there was no clear time of onset, he was not thrombolysed for the presumed stroke syndrome but was admitted for further assessment.

The night after admission he became less alert, weaker in the left leg and complained of severe left leg pain. Assessment at this point revealed new ataxia in the left upper limb, a cold, pale left lower limb and the absence of the left dorsalis pedis pulse. A repeat ECG demonstrated acute T wave inversion in the inferior leads. An urgent CT abdomen with femoral and iliac CT angiogram revealed apparent thrombus adherent to the posterior wall of the abdominal aorta, apparent thrombus in the left superior femoral artery and multiple bilateral renal infarcts. CT head demonstrated multiple acute infarcts located in both cerebellar hemispheres, left occipital lobe and thalamus, right centrum semiovale and right frontal lobe (see below Fig. 24.1):

Urgent transthoracic echocardiography showed apical hypokinesia with an ejection fraction of 40–45% but no valvular vegetations, and no intracardiac thrombi or mass.

He was treated urgently with a left femoral angioplasty plus embolectomy, a left lower limb fasciotomy and also for suspected acute myocardial infarction with heparin and dual antiplatelet agents. A few days later a transoesphageal echocardiogram showed a mobile irregular mass attached to the left side of the interatrial septum and the histology from the femoral embolectomy specimen was reviewed. The appearances were consistent with embolic fragments from an atrial myxoma (Fig. 24.2).

Although his left leg was successfully revascularised, the toes of his left foot became necrotic and subsequently mummified. His progress over the following weeks was also hampered by a series of chest infections and severe infection at the fasciotomy site which required debridement and subsequent skin grafting. After 2 months of treatment for these complications he was finally fit enough to undergo excision of the atrial mass which was carried out via a midline sternotomy and inter-

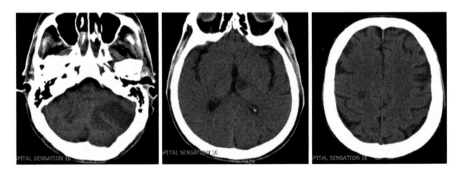

Fig. 24.1 CT head demonstrating acute infarcts in multiple vascular territories

Fig. 24.2 Transoesophageal echocardiogram (one selected image) showing an irregular mass attached to the left side of the interatrial septum (*white arrow*). The mass does not involve the cardiac valves and its echodensity is in keeping with myxoma rather than intracardiac thrombus

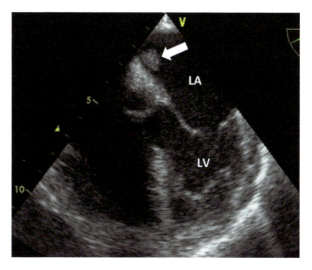

atrial septal approach. Subsequent histological examination confirmed atrial myxoma. The post operative course was uneventful and he was referred to his local stroke unit for rehabilitation.

Discussion

Atrial myxoma arise from the multipotential mesenchymal cells of the endocardium and are left-sided in approximately 85% of cases. Most originate in the limbus fossae ovalis but 10% are found in other regions including the anterior and posterior walls of the atria or the atrial appendages. The tumour is characterised by a gelatinous mass which is round, oval or polypoid in shape, often pedunculated, and is white, yellowish or brown in colour. The surface may be smooth or lobulated and often has adherent thrombus. The incidence is 0.5/million people per year, usually occurring in the 5th or 6th decade and it affects twice as many women as men. In 7% of cases a genetic cause is found, the most common being the Carney complex of cardiac, cutaneous and endocrine abnormalities due to a mutation in the PRKAR1 gene on long arm chromosome 17 [1, 2].

Ischaemic stroke from embolic occlusion of the middle cerebral artery is the most common presentation of atrial myxoma although it is a very rare cause of stroke overall (<1%). Other reported neurological manifestations include seizures (due to ischaemic stroke, haemorrhage from myxoma-related aneurysm, or cortical metastasis), visual loss (due to retinal artery involvement) and paraplegia (due to spinal cord infarction or infrarenal aortic embolus). Associated symptoms due to obstruction of the mitral valve are common at presentation and include dyspnoea, palpitations, dizziness, cardiac failure or even sudden cardiac death. Myxomas have been demonstrated to produce numerous growth factors and cytokines (including vascular endothelial growth factor) and in particular lead to an increased expression of the inflammatory cytokine, interleukin-6. This is thought to be the cause of the associated constitutional symptoms which occur in a large proportion of cases i.e. myalgia, arthralgia, weight loss, fatigue, fever, Raynaud's phenomenon, and finger clubbing [1].

The diagnosis is often made in the context of a patient with embolic stroke, when the tumour is visualised on either transthoracic or transoesophageal echocardiography. Other imaging modalites which can detect the intracardiac mass include dye ventriculography and cardiac CT. The neuroradiological features are those of embolic cerebral infarction (simultaneous or sequential strokes in different arterial territories) and angiography may demonstrate focal dilatations consistent with fusiform aneurysms. Myxoma-related aneurysms are thought to be caused by direct invasion of the vessel wall by tumour metastases rather than blood-flow dynamics (hence their fusiform rather than saccular shape). Blood tests may reveal evidence of an acute phase response with anaemia, raised CRP and ESR plus hypergammaglobulinaemia [1, 3].

There is little evidence to guide the acute management of patients with atrial myxoma who present with acute stroke. Given the frequent finding of thombus combined with myxoma in peripheral emboli, treatment with intravenous rTPA would seem logical (and in fact the myxoma is often undiagnosed until well after thrombolysis has been given). Balanced against this is the theoretical increased risk of post-thrombolysis haemorrhage from occult tumour emboli and microaneurysms. In numerous case reports, intravenous thrombolysis has been used successfully, or at least has not resulted in a significant clinical deterioration [4–8], though severe intracerebral haemorrhage was reported in one early case [9] and the risk of haemorrhage in one small series was higher in those over 70 years old [10]. In stroke patients with known myxoma, treatment with intraarterial thrombolysis and/or a clot retrieval device may be more effective than standard intravenous thrombolysis [6]. The curative treatment for atrial myxoma is surgical resection, following which annual echocardiographic assessment is recommended for 3–4 years in sporadic cases and lifelong in Carney complex patients. The recurrence rate after excision in cases of sporadic atrial myxoma is 5% though the long-term prognosis is good, with an average 20-year survival rate of 85% [1].

Key Clinical Learning Points
1. Atrial myxoma is a rare cause of stroke but should always be considered in the differential diagnosis of embolic cerebral infarction, or of stroke in a young patient
2. There is little strong evidence to guide hyperacute management in cases of acute stroke and known myxoma though numerous case reports suggest that intravenous thrombolysis is generally safe and often effective
3. The curative treatment for myxoma is surgical excision but in the pre-operative period warfarin or aspirin should be used to protect against thromboembolism from the tumour surface or from thrombus-rich tumour fragments

Key Radiological Learning Points

1. The main neuroradiological findings in atrial myxoma are embolic cerebral infarction, intracranial aneurysms and intracerebral or subarachnoid haemorrhage
2. Diagnosis can depend on good quality transoesphageal echocardiography to visualise the tumour and to distinguish it from other sources of cardioembolic stroke

References

1. Lee VH, Connolly HM, Brown Jr RD. Central nervous system manifestations of cardiac myxoma. Arch Neurol. 2007;64(8):1115–20.
2. Wold LE, Lie JT. Cardiac myxomas: a clinicopathologic profile. Am J Pathol. 1980;101: 219–40.
3. Novendstern SL, Silliman SL, Booth P. Cerebrovascular complications of atrial myxoma. Hosp Phys. 2001;3:39–42.
4. Acampa M, Tassi R, Guideri F, et al. Safety of intravenous thrombolysis in ischemic stroke caused by left atrial myxoma. Curr Drug Saf. 2011;6(5):343–5.
5. Ibrahim M, Iliescu C, Safi HJ, et al. Biatrial myxoma and cerebral ischemia successfully treated with intravenous thrombolytic therapy and surgical resection. Tex Heart Inst J. 2008;35: 193–5.
6. Kohno N, Kawakami Y, Hamada C, et al. Cerebral embolism associated with left atrial myxoma that was treated with thrombolytic therapy. Case Rep Neurol. 2012;4:38–42.
7. Nagy CD, Levy M, Mulhearn TJ, et al. Safe and effective intravenous thrombolysis for acute ischemic stroke caused by left atrial myxoma. J Stroke Cerebrovasc Dis. 2009;18:398–402.
8. Sun MC, Tai HC, Lee CH. Intravenous thrombolysis for embolic stroke due to cardiac myxoma. Case Rep Neurol. 2011;3:21–6.
9. Chong JY, Vraniak P, Etienne M, et al. Intravenous thrombolytic treatment of acute ischemic stroke associated with left atrial myxoma: a case report. J Stroke Cerebrovasc Dis. 2005;14: 39–41.
10. Ong CT. Intravenous thrombolysis associated with a high risk of hemorrhagic transformation in ischemic stroke patients with cardiac myxoma and over 70 years of age. Neurol Asia. 2012;17(3):193–7.

Chapter 25
Sleep Disordered Breathing and Stroke

Ari Manuel and Sumanjit K. Gill

Clinical History

A 64-year-old right-handed lady was admitted to hospital with the sudden onset of dizziness, vomiting, slurred speech, clumsiness of the right arm and veering to the right.

She had a history of a previous left hemiparesis from which she had fully recovered, atrial fibrillation, hypertension, hypercholesterolaemia and a basal cell carcinoma of the nose. She was a non-smoker. Her BMI was 28.

She was on warfarin but her INR was poorly controlled and she had frequently been in the subtherapeutic range. She lived with her husband and was independent in activities of daily living.

Examination

Neurological examination revealed dysarthria, horizontal nystagmus to the right and right upper limb ataxia. There was no Horner's syndrome or sensory deficit. There were no deficits in the lower limbs. She was able to put names to familiar objects and could draw a clock face. Cardiovascular examination revealed an irregularly irregular pulse with a rate of 85 beats per minute, an elevated blood pressure at 164/126 mmHg and no detectable murmurs. Her National Institutes of Health Stroke Score (NIHSS) was 2.

A. Manuel, MBBS, MRCP, BSc, DipLATHE
Oxford Sleep Unit, Oxford University Hospitals NHS Trust, Oxford, Oxfordshire, UK
e-mail: arimanuel1979@yahoo.co.uk

S.K. Gill, BSc Hons, MBBS, MRCP (✉)
Education Unit, National Hospital for Neurology and Neurosurgery,
UCL Institute of Neurology, London, UK
e-mail: sumanjit.gill@nhs.net

© Springer-Verlag London 2015
S.K. Gill et al. (eds.), *Stroke Medicine: Case Studies from Queen Square*,
DOI 10.1007/978-1-4471-6705-1_25

Investigations

Blood tests showed a sub-therapeutic INR of 1.3 but were otherwise normal. The haemoglobin and haematocrit were normal.

A CT brain revealed a mature infarct in the right frontal region, small vessel disease and bilateral basal ganglia calcification, none of which were thought to account for her presentation.

Clinical Progress

As her NIHSS was very low a decision was made not to thrombolyse. Reloading with warfarin was commenced. No progression of deficit was recorded within the next 36 hours.

However on day two of her inpatient stay, she was observed to be coughing on eating. She failed a swallow screen and she was re scanned to look for any extension of her infarct.

An MRI with diffusion-weighted imaging confirmed an acute infarct involving the right cerebellar hemisphere medially and the posterior aspect of the right medulla in typical right PICA territory (Fig. 25.1).

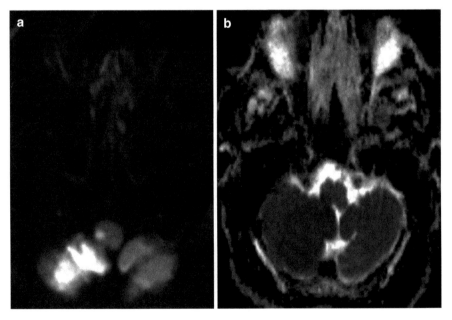

Fig. 25.1 Diffusion weighted B1000 image (*left*) and ADC map (*right*) showing acute restriction in the inferior cerebellar hemisphere and posterolateral medullary infarction, typical of an acute right PICA territory infarct

Warfarin loading continued but over the following days she became confused overnight with variable oxygen saturations and the nursing staff witnessed apnoeic episodes up to 15 seconds in duration. Her daytime arterial blood gases were normal. She was not on any respiratory depressant drugs.

She went on to have overnight oximetry which was highly suggestive of obstructive sleep apnoea (OSA). She was recorded having an oxygen desaturation index (ODI) of 35/per hour. She was commenced on continuous positive air pressure machine (CPAP) and although initially she struggled to use the device, by the time of discharge she was successfully using it most of the night.

Her history was revisited and revealed a history of snoring, daytime somnolence and witnessed apnoeas to support the diagnosis of obstructive sleep apnoea and her Epworth Sleepiness Score (ESS) was 12 (Normal < 9) She continued rehabilitation on the stroke unit and her swallowing recovered such that she could tolerate a soft diet.

An Echocardiogram performed confirmed moderate global hypokinesia but no evidence of thrombus. A decision was made to switch her anticoagulation from warfarin to rivaroxaban 20 mg once daily for her atrial fibrillation in view of her problems with managing a variably dosed drug.

She was discharged home after a 1-month inpatient stay with a plan to continue using cPAP overnight.

Discussion

Sleep-related breathing disturbances (SDB) are frequently under diagnosed in stroke patients. SDB, presenting with obstructive, central, or mixed apnoeas, are present in 50–70% of stroke patients [1].

There is strong evidence from large epidemiological studies that obstructive sleep apnoea (OSA) contributes to the development of stroke [1, 2] partly through the association of known risk factors for stroke such as hypertension [3] and diabetes. It is very important to exclude OSA when secondary polycythaemia is present, which can be marginal (in terms of red cell count/Hb/haematocrit) in many patients. Patients with stroke and polycythaemia need urgent venesection.

For clinical screening, the Epworth score is designed to assess the degree of daytime somnolence. Patients suspected of suffering with OSA undergo a sleep study, which records the number of periods of apnoeas or hypopneas overnight. This is used to aid the physician to classify OSA into mild, moderate or severe.

After stroke, severe OSA increases the risk of recurrence and mortality. OSA is present in 44–72% of poststroke patients [4] and probably promotes further functional impairment through intermittent nocturnal hypoxia, reduced cerebral perfusion, and fragmented sleep. It can also impede progress with rehabilitation by causing daytime fatigue and reduced attention [5].

OSA is seldom considered during the poststroke period despite evidence that managing OSA may benefit patients with stroke. It is difficult to isolate OSA as a risk factor as it is strongly associated with vascular disease. However, the literature does support that OSA constitutes an independent risk. However, two key clinical diagnostic criteria, excessive daytime sleepiness (EDS) and obesity, do not appear to be prevalent in patients poststroke. For example, Bassetti et al. [6] reported that 26 of 152 patients with stroke had severe OSA with an AHI ≥30, but their mean EDS score of 6.8 and BMI of 27.9 kg/m^2 indicated that they were generally neither subjectively sleepy nor obese. However, post stroke fatigue is commonly seen and it may be difficult to differentiate from the somnolence.

CPAP treatment should be reserved for patients with severe obstructive SDB, daytime symptoms (e.g., sleepiness), or a high cardiovascular risk profile.

It is vital that the need for CPAP in the acute phase is assessed by taking blood gases as hypercapnia causes a dilatation of cerebral blood vessels in normal areas of brain diverting blood from the infarcted area – this is termed 'Reversed Robin Hood Syndrome' [7]. This can lead to a higher risk of recurrent stroke.

Existing studies provide sufficient data to establish obstructive SDB as a negative predictor of all-cause mortality and recurrent vascular events following stroke or TIA [8]. The ability of CPAP treatment to lower the risk of serious adverse outcomes after stroke remains controversial [7].

Key Clinical Learning Points
1. Sleep disordered breathing is often present but overlooked in stroke patients
2. Hypoventilation can impair recovery and limit the ability to participate in rehabilitation
3. Obstructive sleep apnoea is strongly linked with TIA and stroke
4. It is screened for by using the Epworth score and diagnosed with a sleep study to assess the number of instances of apnoea and hypopnoea
5. Patients with Central Sleep Apnoea may require different forms of ventilatory support and those with OSA should be considered for treatment with CPAP

References

1. Arzt M, Young T, Finn L, et al. Association of sleep-disordered breathing and the occurrence of stroke. Am J Respir Crit Care Med. 2005;172:1447–51.
2. Munoz R, Duran-Cantolla J, Martinez-Vila E, et al. Severe sleep apnea and risk of ischemic stroke in the elderly. Stroke. 2006;37:2317–21.
3. Becker HF, Jerrentrup A, Ploch T, et al. Effect of nasal continuous positive airway pressure treatment on blood pressure in patients with obstructive sleep apnea. Circulation. 2003;107:68–73.
4. Kaneko Y, Hajek VE, Zivanovic V, et al. Relationship of sleep apnea to functional capacity and length of hospitalization following stroke. Sleep. 2003;26:293–7.
5. Good DC, Henkle JQ, Gelber D, et al. Sleep-disordered breathing and poor functional outcome after stroke. Stroke. 1996;27:252–9.

6. Bassetti C, Aldrich MS, Chervin RD, et al. Sleep apnea in patients with transient ischemic attack and stroke: a prospective study of 59 patients. Neurology. 1996;47:1167–73.
7. Palazzo P, Balucani C, Barlinn K, et al. Association of reversed Robin Hood syndrome with risk of stroke recurrence. Neurology. 2010;75(22):2003–8.
8. Birkbak J, Clark AJ, Rod NH. The effect of sleep disordered breathing on the outcome of stroke and transient ischemic attack: a systematic review. J Clin Sleep Med. 2014;10(1): 103–8.

Chapter 26
A Possible Remedy for Post Stroke Confusion

Raja Farhat Shoaib, Anthony O'Brien, Thaya Loganathan, Shaun Ude, Devesh Sinha, James R. Brown, and Paul Guyler

Clinical History

A 73-year-old lady was admitted to the acute stroke unit with two discreet episodes of right-sided weakness, sensory loss and expressive dysphasia. Each lasted 42 minutes with complete resolution. Her past medical history included a partial right MCA syndrome, giant cell arteritis with consequent blindness of the right eye and post-stroke seizures. She was taking clopidogrel, levetiracetam and a statin. She was living alone and her modified Rankin score was zero. She used to smoke in past but stopped 35 years previously.

Examination and Investigations

On admission her neurological examination was unremarkable apart from confusion with a Montreal Cognitive Assessment (MOCA) score of 9/30. She was diagnosed clinically with a high-risk transient ischaemic attack (ABCD² score was 5) and admitted. However, an MRI scan of her brain showed a small left posterior parietal infarction on DWI (Fig. 26.1). A carotid Doppler ultrasound scan showed a very high flow velocity in the left internal carotid artery (suggesting 90% stenosis)

R.F. Shoaib, MRCPS (✉) • A. O'Brien, MRCP • T. Loganathan, MRCP • S. Ude, MRCP
D. Sinha, MRCP • P. Guyler, MRCP
Acute Stroke Medicine, Southend University Hospital, Southend on sea, Essex, UK
e-mail: shoaibrf@hotmail.com

J.R. Brown, FRCS
Department of Vascular Surgery, Southend University Hospital, Southend on sea, Essex, UK

© Springer-Verlag London 2015
S.K. Gill et al. (eds.), *Stroke Medicine: Case Studies from Queen Square*,
DOI 10.1007/978-1-4471-6705-1_26

163

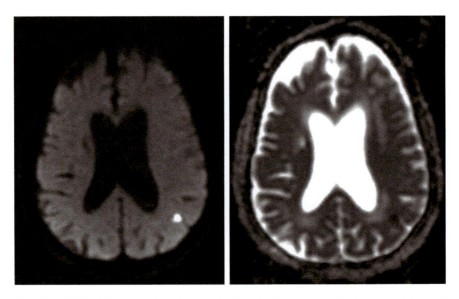

Fig. 26.1 B1000 diffusion weighted image (*left*) and ADC map (*right*) show small focus if restricted diffusion in the left parietal lobe in keeping with an acute infarct

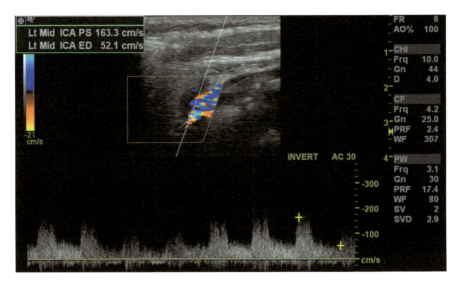

Fig. 26.2 Image from carotid doppler ultrasound study showing increased ICA PS (Peak systolic) velocity

and complete occlusion of the right internal carotid artery (Fig. 26.2). A CT angiogram (CTA) was performed and showed concordant results with a heavily calcified left carotid bulb causing 90% stenosis (Fig. 26.3).

Fig. 26.3 Image from CT angiogram study showing calcified plaque narrowing the left ICA (*white arrow*)

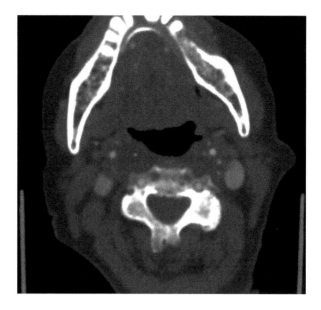

Clinical Progress

During her admission, she became very agitated at night with visual hallucinations and verbal aggression. Septic and metabolic screens were normal. Her confusion was considered disproportionate to the size of the infarction. Her case was discussed at a neurovascular multidisciplinary meeting and carotid endarterectomy was planned, which she underwent on day 7 of her admission.

Postoperatively her MOCA improved from 9 pre-op to 20/30 and nocturnal confusion resolved. Her medications were optimised and she was discharged to her usual place of residence (Fig. 26.1).

Discussion

Vascular cognitive impairment has several different causes [1] but the clinical co-relation between carotid artery disease and cognitive impairment was first proposed by Fisher, based on necropsy case [2]. He postulated that carotid occlusive disease can produce dementia and cognitive impairment through hypoperfusion alone and restoration of blood flow can improve condition.

Carotid artery stenosis is responsible for 20% of anterior circulation infarction. Silent cerebral micro-infarction due to emboli originating from carotid atheroma do not manifest as frank stroke [3]. The Rotterdam study showed that silent infarction picked up on MRI scan in elderly people can double the risk of dementia and lead to decline in cognitive function [4]. In addition, patients with silent infarction are at higher risk of additional small infarcts or even symptomatic major ischaemic strokes [5]. High-grade carotid stenosis is associated with not only altered perfusion and diffusion but also neurocognitive impairment. This is most likely due to white matter degeneration. As stroke and silent ischaemia may be a cause of cognitive decline and early dementia in the elderly [6, 7], it is reasonable to hypothesize that symptomatic patients have a greater burden of ischaemic changes than asymptomatic patients and consequently are at greater risk of cognitive impairment [3].

Carotid revascularisation leads to improved cerebral blood flow, which can result in improvement in cognitive function [8]. This potential benefit would be derived by all patients irrespective of method of revascularisation either CEA or carotid stenting. However, each procedure can result in transient reduction in cerebral blood flow during carotid clamping or deployment of a protection device, which becomes evident by flattening of EEG trace when cerebral blood flow is below 18 ml/100 g per minute [9].

Most of the studies that have evaluated cognitive function before and after carotid endarterectomy have shown improvement. However, there are no clear recommendations about endarterectomy in treating cognitive deficit in otherwise asymptomatic patients [10]. One study has shown that symptomatic patients especially with minor stroke are more likely to show post-operative improvement in cognitive function than patients with less severe symptoms [3]. To our knowledge, this is the first case report describing full resolution of nocturnal confusion following endarterectomy.

Key Clinical Learning Points
1. Carotid stenosis can be associated with vascular cognitive impairment through either causing silent strokes or by causing hypoperfusion
2. It maybe possible to slow this process by revascularising the carotid artery
3. Delirium is possible post-stroke especially in the acute phase and possible causes e.g. sepsis or electrolyte imbalance should be explored

References

1. Bowler JV. The concept of vascular cognitive impairment. J Neurol Sci. 2002;203:11–5.
2. Fisher C. Senile dementia – a new explanation of its causation. Arch Neurol. 1951;65:1–7.
3. Baracchini C, Mazzalai F, Gruppo M, et al. Carotid endarterectomy protects elderly patients from cognitive decline. Surgery. 2012;151(1):99–106.
4. Vermeer SE, Prins ND, Den Heijer T, et al. Silent brain infarcts and risk of dementia and cognitive decline. N Engl J Med. 2003;348:1215–22.
5. Bernick C, Kuller L, Dulberg C. Silent MRI infarcts and risk of future strokes. The endovascular health study. Neurology. 2001;57:1222–9.

6. Desmond DW, Moroney JT, Sano M, et al. Incidence of dementia after stroke. Stroke. 2002;363:1491–502.
7. Norris JW, Zhu CZ. Silent stroke and carotid stenosis. Stroke. 1992;23:483–5.
8. Marshall RS, Lazer RM, Pile-Spellman J, et al. Recovery of brain function during induced cerebral hypoperfusion. Brain. 2001;124:1208–17.
9. Marshall RS. The functional relevance of cerebral hemodynamics: Why blood flow matters to injured and recovering brain. Curr Opin Neurol. 2004;17:705–9.
10. Demarin V, Zavoreo I, Kes VB. Carotid artery disease and cognitive impairment. J Neurol Sci. 2012;322:107–11.

Chapter 27
A Headache with a Difference

Sumanjit K. Gill, Stefanie Christina Robert, and Anish Bahra

Clinical History

A 45-year-old right-handed female shop worker presented to the emergency department with a 4-hour history of severe unilateral headache. She described loss of vision on her right side that occurred simultaneously with the onset of the headache. She reported that the headache was severe and throbbing in character. Her husband reported that her speech had changed and that she had become slow to respond.

She had a past medical history of bilateral sensorineural hearing loss, diagnosed in 1996. She had no vascular risk factors, and was not taking any medication.

Examination

She was alert and orientated. Her temperature was 37.9 °C. Examination revealed that she had a right homonymous hemianopia. She was dysphasic with both a receptive and expressive component. She did not have any limb weakness. Her left

S.K. Gill, BSc Hons, MBBS, MRCP (✉)
Education Unit, National Hospital for Neurology and Neurosurgery, UCL Institute of Neurology, London, UK
e-mail: sumanjit.gill@nhs.net

S.C. Robert, MD, MRCP, FFICM
Intensive Care Unit, Homerton University Hospital, London, UK

A. Bahra, FRCP, MD
Department of Neurology, Bartshealth, Whipps Cross Hospital, London, UK

Department of Neurology, National Hospital for Neurology and Neurosurgery, London, UK

© Springer-Verlag London 2015
S.K. Gill et al. (eds.), *Stroke Medicine: Case Studies from Queen Square*,
DOI 10.1007/978-1-4471-6705-1_27

plantar response was upgoing. Her chest was clear and her oxygen saturations 95% on air. Her heart sounds were normal with no added sounds. Her blood pressure was elevated at 175/65 mmHg. Skin and joint examination were normal.

Investigations and Clinical Progress

Routine blood tests including CRP were in the normal range. Her ECG showed her to be in sinus rhythm. Initial CT head was reported as normal. She had a lumbar puncture and protein, glucose and cell count were all within normal limits. She was started on high dose aspirin.

A few hours into her admission the patient had 2 generalised tonic clonic seizures in quick succession. These were terminated with diazepam followed by a phenytoin infusion. A florid rash occurred with phenytoin, which was discontinued and replaced with valproate. However, the seizures recurred on valproate and phenobarbitone was substituted achieving seizure control.

Repeat CT and MRI imaging was subsequently performed demonstrating an acute right hemisphere infarct (Figs. 27.1 and 27.2). The infarct was considered unusual in that it spans two conventional vascular territories (right MCA and PCA) and other unusual conditions were considered. Blood analysis demonstrated an A to G substitution at nucleotide position 3243 of her mitochondrial DNA making the diagnosis of Mitochondrial Encephalopathy and Lactic Acidosis with Stroke Like Episodes (MELAS).

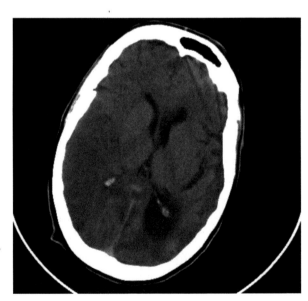

Fig. 27.1 Unenhanced axial CT image showing large area of acute infarction posteriorly in the right hemisphere involving temporal/parietal and occipital lobes

Fig. 27.2 Axial T2 weighted image, showing infarction in a similar distribution

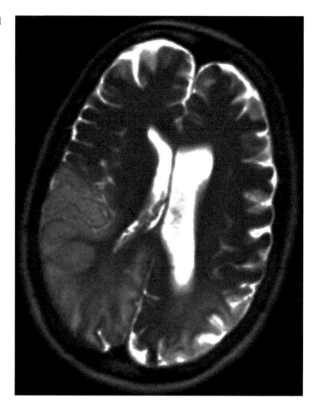

Discussion

MELAS is a mitochondrial disorder which commonly manifests between the ages of 20 and 40 years and follows a relapsing and remitting course. The commonest presentation is with a stroke-like episode and there is an association with sensori-neural deafness. It also causes seizures, migraine-like headaches, lactic acidosis, myopathy and dementia. The diagnosis is confirmed with blood leucocyte analysis. The most common mutation is $A \rightarrow G$ 3243 – seen in 80% of cases. Another is $T \rightarrow C$ at position 3271. There can be variation in its clinical presentation due to the phenomenon of heteroplasmy; the proportion of affected mitochondria determines the nature and severity of the clinical phenotype. Diffusion weighted MR imaging is sensitive for the stroke like lesions in the acute phase. Muscle biopsy classically shows ragged red fibres [1, 2].

The pathogenesis of stroke-like lesions in MELAS remains unclear. The lesions are often seen in the occipital lobe and typically do not conform to a defined vascular territories. Unlike conventional 'arterial strokes' they often resolve rapidly. Current opinion supports a metabolic rather than a vascular cause [1].

The only success in the treatment of stroke-like episodes has been with the use of L-arginine infusions, which has been shown to resolve the episode within

30 minutes. When followed by oral supplementation there may be a significant decrease in both the frequency and severity of stroke like episodes [1].

There may be a link between valproate and the exacerbation of seizures in patients with MELAS, based on previous case reports [2–4]. The mechanism of this remains unclear, although it is not an isolated phenomenon – the use of valproate in other mitochondrial diseases (e.g: those involving POLG1 mutations) also has adverse effects.

Statins should also be avoided in patients with MELAS as they may worsen pre-existing myopathy.

MELAS is one of several single gene disorders, which have stroke as a prominent feature in their clinical presentation [5, 6]. A table is given below with some of the commoner of these diseases with the most common contributory gene defects. This list is by no means exhaustive, but provides the main genetic differential diagnosis when investigating a more unusual presentation or a younger patient with stroke (Table 27.1).

Table 27.1 Single gene defects associated with stroke [5, 6]

Example	Gene defect	Diagnosis	Mechanism
Atrial myxoma Familial arrhythmias and cardiomyopathies	A variety	Electrophysiological testing Cardiac imaging/ biopsy	Cardioembolic
Homocystinuria	Any one of a possible 150 mutations in the cystathionine-beta gene (CBS) located on chromosome 21	Plasma and urine levels	Metabolic: prothrombotic
Protein S deficiency Protein C deficiency Antithrombin III deficiency	PROS1 gene mutation PROC gene on chr 2 Point mutations of the antithrombin gene	Plasma assay	Prothrombotic: Venous thromboembolism that can traverse a patent foramen ovale to cause arterial stroke
CADASIL	Mutation on Notch 3 on chromosome 19	Blood DNA analysis	Small and medium arterial vessel disease
MELAS	80% Single base mutation A → G 3243	leucocyte DNA analysis	Metabolic: mitochondrial disease
Marfan's syndrome	Defect in fibrillin gene: FBN-1 on chromosome 15	Clinical diagnosis in most cases	Arterial Dissection
Ehlers-Danlos syndrome	Mutations most commonly in any one of the following ADAMTS2, COL1A1, COL1A2, COL3A1, COL5A1, COL5A2, PLOD1	Clinical diagnosis in most cases: Joint hypermobility and laxity as measured on the Beighton scale	Arterial dissection

Table 27.1 (Continued)

Example	Gene defect	Diagnosis	Mechanism
Familial hemiplegic migraine	Mutation in either one of the CACNA1A, ATP1A2 or SCN1A genes	Clinical as not all mutations have been identified	Channelopathy of the voltage gated calcium channel leading to increased susceptibility to decreased blood flow
Fabry's disease	Galactosidase alpha gene – GLA on chromosome 22	Leukocyte DNA analysis of alpha-galactosidase activity Isolation of mutations in the GLA gene	Vessel ectasia Large vessel occlusive disease Small vessel disease

Key Clinical Learning Points
1. MELAS is a mitochondrial disorder presenting with stroke like episodes
2. The only evidence-based treatment is L-arginine infusion
3. Statins should be avoided in these patients as they may exacerbate the associated myopathy
4. Valproate should be avoided in these patients as the may provoke seizures

Key Radiological Learning Points
1. The 'ischaemic' lesions seen on imaging in MELAS patients do not conform to conventional vascular territories
2. Lesions are often seen in the occipital lobes
3. Diffusion weighted imaging demonstrates matched defects which may resolve rapidly

References

1. Koga Y, Akita Y, Nishioka J, et al. MELAS and l arginine therapy. Mitochondrion. 2007;7: 133–9.
2. Lam CW, Lau CH, Williams JC, et al. Mitochondrial Myopathy, Encephalopathy, Lactic Acidosis and Stroke Like Episodes (MELAS) triggered by valproate therapy. Eur J Pediatr. 1997;156(7):562–4.
3. Lin CM, Thajeb P. Valproic acid aggravates epilepsy due to MELAS in a patient with an A3243G mutation of mitochondrial DNA. Metab Brain Dis. 2007;22(1):105–9.
4. Hsu YC, Yang FC, Perng CL, et al. Adult onset of Mitochondrial Myopathy, Encephalopathy, Lactic Acidosis and Stroke Like Episodes (MELAS) syndrome presenting as an acute meningoencephalitis: a case report. J Emerg Med. 2012;43(3):e163–6.
5. Hassan A, Markus HS. Genetics and ischaemic stroke. Brain. 2000;123:1784–812.
6. Sharma P, Yadav S, Meschia JF. Genetics of ischaemic stroke. J Neurol Neurosurg Psychiatry. 2013;84:1302–8. doi:10.1136/jnnp-2012-304834.

Chapter 28
An Alternative Solution to a Difficult Problem

Kelvin Kuan Huei Ng

Clinical History

A 64-year-old gentleman was found by his wife slumped to the right side, unable to speak with ongoing epistaxis at about 6 o'clock in the morning. He was last seen well before going to bed just before midnight the previous day. He was accompanied by his wife to the emergency room. She reported he had intermittent epistaxis for the past week and had to stop taking aspirin prescribed for paroxysmal atrial fibrillation.

He had a diagnosis of hereditary haemorrhagic telangiectasia and usually required iron supplementation and regular blood transfusion for recurrent epistaxis despite embolization and surgical ligation of his nasal vessels. He had hypertension and a stable type B thoracic aorta dissection and an abdominal aortic aneurysm under routine surveillance. He was not noted to have any other significant vascular malformations elsewhere. He did not smoke or drink alcohol. He had previously had an uncomplicated resection of a left adrenal tumour around 7 years ago.

His medications included pantoprazole, irbesartan, hydrochlorothiazide, atorvastatin and metoprolol. He had been prescribed aspirin 81 mg once daily but took it only intermittently due to his recurrent epistaxis.

Examination

On arrival to the emergency room, he was alert and cooperative. He had right sided facial weakness sparing the forehead and dense right sided hemiplegia. He had predominantly expressive dysphasia but no neglect. Sensation was intact.

K.K.H. Ng, MBBS
Stroke Neurology Department, Hamilton General Hospital, Hamilton, ON, Canada
e-mail: kelvin.ng@phri.ca

© Springer-Verlag London 2015   175
S.K. Gill et al. (eds.), *Stroke Medicine: Case Studies from Queen Square*,
DOI 10.1007/978-1-4471-6705-1_28

Cardiovascular examination demonstrated a soft ejection systolic murmur loudest over the precordium. Respiratory and abdominal examination were unremarkable apart from a well healed surgical scar.

Investigations and Clinical Progress[1]

Routine blood work on admission was within normal range apart from a normocytic anaemia (haemoglobin of 87 g/L). ECG showed no obvious abnormality and he was in sinus rhythm.

CT Scan of Head on Admission is Shown (Fig. 28.1)

Carotid Doppler ultrasound showed no evidence of significant stenosis in the extra-cranial segment of both internal carotid arteries. Twenty-four hour Holter ECG monitor showed sinus rhythm with frequent short runs of atrial tachycardia but no sustained atrial fibrillation.

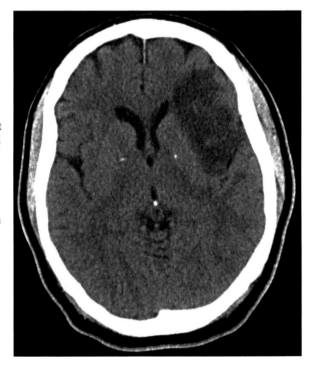

Fig. 28.1 There is significant hypodensity in the left frontal region encompassing most of the insular ribbon and external capsule with mild effacement and mass effect. There is a small amount of petechial haemorrhage within the infarct zone. This cortically based infarct was thought to be due to a proximal embolic source. In the absence of significant cervical carotid artery disease, a cardiogenic embolus from paroxysmal atrial fibrillation was suspected

Both the transthoracic and transoesophageal echocardiogram demonstrated the old type B aortic dissection in the descending aorta distal to the left subclavian artery. There was severe biatrial enlargement but no significant valve disease with preserved left ventricular function.

After completing the investigations for the underlying aetiology of the stroke, he was diagnosed with likely embolic stroke secondary to paroxysmal atrial fibrillation. His CHA_2DS_2-VaSc was 4.

He recovered from his initial stroke with minimal residual weakness in his right arm and leg. He continued to have residual mild expressive dysphasia.

Taking into account his propensity to bleed, he was restarted on aspirin but continued to have further nose bleeds requiring inpatient blood transfusions. As he was intolerant of antithrombotic agents, he was referred to the cardiologists and later the cardiothoracic surgeons for consideration of left atrial excision for stroke prophylaxis. Following a lengthy discussion with the patient and his family, he went on to have an open surgical excision of his left atrial appendage for secondary stroke prevention.

He had a further period of rehabilitation post-operatively and was eventually discharged home without antiplatelets or anticoagulants.

Discussion

Hereditary haemorrhagic telangiectasia is a rare disorder composed of a triad of mucocutaneous telangiectasia, recurrent epistaxis or gastrointestinal haemorrhage and a family history of the disorder. The condition is inherited in a Mendelian dominant manner. In the central nervous system, vascular anomalies include telangiectasia, arteriovenous malformations, aneurysms and rarely, carotid-cavernous fistulae. Pulmonary venous fistulae can be responsible for paradoxical embolism resulting in stroke or transient ischaemic attack. Hypoxia due to significant right to left shunting can result in mental obtundation and polycythaemia. Rarely, air embolism or portosystemic encephalopathy can occur.

Whilst arteriovenous malformations in hereditary haemorrhagic telangiectasia can be associated with stroke, patients can also have 'classical' risk factors for stroke. Unfortunately, the patients' propensity to bleed may pose therapeutic challenges [1].

In this case, the patient also has atrial fibrillation, a common, preventable cause of disabling stroke. The left atrial appendage is well recognised as the source for thromboembolism in atrial fibrillation. Pharmacological therapy with antiplatelets or oral anticoagulants are effective at reducing the risk of stroke in patients with atrial fibrillation but the benefit of antiplatelets are attenuated with increasing age [2]. The novel selective oral anticoagulants such as dabigatran, rivaroxaban and apixaban are at least as effective as warfarin but appear safer with lower rates of intracranial haemorrhage. Based on the AVERROES trial, the risk of bleeding on apixaban is similar to aspirin [3].

If long term antiplatelet agents or oral anticoagulation are not tolerated, percutaneous left atrial appendage occlusion can be considered. There are several devices at various levels of development at the moment (AMPLATZER Cardiac plug, LARIAT Suture Delivery Device, WATCHMAN Left Atrial Appendage System). The only published randomised controlled trial of an implanted percutaneous device (WATCHMAN; Aritech Inc., Plymouth, Minnesota) found the device to be at least as effective as long term warfarin therapy for preventing stroke in selected populations [4, 5]. However, in the PROTECT-AF trial, patients were on warfarin for at least 45 days after device implantation before going on to dual antiplatelet agents for 6 months and finally aspirin monotherapy thereafter. The study compared the WATCHMAN device in addition to a complex antithrombotic regime against long-term warfarin in a predominantly low risk, primary prevention population. Unfortunately, PROTECT-AF did not compare the WATCHMAN device against patients deemed unsuitable for long-term warfarin, a population which best describes our patient.

In addition, our patient did not tolerate long-term aspirin and was at high risk of further events unlike the population in PROTECT-AF.

Open surgical left atrial amputation or occlusion can be considered in selected cases. Evidence is limited to predominantly retrospective case series in patients following coronary artery bypass grafts or mitral valve replacements. The LAAOS III is currently ongoing comparing left atrial amputation with aspirin against long term anticoagulation for warfarin following open heart surgery but an early study has been promising [6].

Patients with atrial fibrillation and a CHA_2DS_2-VaSc of 2 or more should be offered oral anticoagulation for stroke prophylaxis. Whilst the novel selective oral anticoagulants appear safer than warfarin, certain groups of patients may not tolerate pharmacological antithrombotic medications. Whilst there exists percutaneous and open surgical options for stroke prophylaxis, conclusive evidence from randomised controlled trials is currently limited.

Key Clinical Learning Points
1. Atrial fibrillation is a common and preventable cause for stroke that is managed with oral anticoagulation in the majority of patients
2. Hereditary haemorrhagic telangiectasia is a rare, inherited vascular disorder that may preclude oral antithrombotics
3. Selected patients may benefit from percutaneous or open surgical left atrial occlusion if oral antithrombotics are contraindicated though conclusive evidence for their benefit remains limited

References

1. Devlin HL, Hosman AE, Shovlin CL. Antiplatelet and anticoagulant agents in hereditary hemorrhagic telangiectasia. N Engl J Med. 2013;368(9):876–8.
2. Van Walraven C, Hart RG, Connolly S, et al. Effect of age on stroke prevention therapy in patients with atrial fibrillation: the atrial fibrillation investigators. Stroke. 2009;40(4):1410–6.
3. Connolly SJ, Eikelboom J, Joyner C, et al. Apixaban in patients with atrial fibrillation. N Engl J Med. 2011;364(9):806–17.
4. Holmes DR, Reddy VY, Turi ZG, et al. Percutaneous closure of the left atrial appendage versus warfarin therapy for prevention of stroke in patients with atrial fibrillation: a randomised non-inferiority trial. Lancet. 2009;374(9689):534–42. Elsevier Ltd.
5. Reddy VY, Doshi SK, Sievert H, et al. Percutaneous left atrial appendage closure for stroke prophylaxis in patients with atrial fibrillation: 2.3-year follow-up of the PROTECT AF (watchman left atrial appendage system for embolic protection in patients with atrial fibrillation) trial. Circulation. 2013;127(6):720–9.
6. Healey JS, Crystal E, Lamy A, et al. Left Atrial Appendage Occlusion Study (LAAOS): results of a randomized controlled pilot study of left atrial appendage occlusion during coronary bypass surgery in patients at risk for stroke. Am Heart J. 2005;150(2):288–93.

Chapter 29
Botox Saves the Day

Laura Flisher, Gerry Christofi, and Rachel Farrell

Clinical History

A 38-year-old right-handed lady was admitted to the neurorehabilitation ward 50 days after the onset of neurological symptoms that came on the day after delivery. She gave a history that during her second pregnancy, she had developed hypertension and pregnancy induced diabetes and subsequently presented with pre-eclampsia requiring emergency caesarean section at 38 weeks gestation. One day later, she developed the acute onset of blurred vision and severe headache. Over the following hours the headache intensified and a left sided ptosis emerged. Initially, she remained alert and oriented with normal speech, but she deteriorated on the third day after delivery with fluctuating level of awareness, speech disturbance and right-sided hemiparesis with facial involvement.

In the past, at the age of 12 she had non-Hodgkin's lymphoma successfully treated and then at the age of 32, she had had a minimally invasive follicular thyroid carcinoma diagnosed. This was treated by thyroidectomy and radioactive iodine ablation. She had developed migraine during a prior pregnancy, age 30, which had subsequently resolved.

L. Flisher, BSs Hons, BSc Hons, HPC, CSP (✉)
Therapies and Rehabilitation, National Hospital for Neurology and Neurosurgery,
London, UK
e-mail: laura.flisher@uclh.nhs.uk

G. Christofi, BSc, PhD, BM BCh, MRCP, MRCP
Neurorehabilitation, National Hospital for Neurology and Neurosurgery, London, UK

R. Farrell, MB BCh, MRCPI, PhD
Neurorehabilitation, National Hospital for Neurology and Neurosurgery, UCLH, London, UK
e-mail: rachel.farrell@uclh.nhs.uk

© Springer-Verlag London 2015
S.K. Gill et al. (eds.), *Stroke Medicine: Case Studies from Queen Square*,
DOI 10.1007/978-1-4471-6705-1_29

Examination

At time of admission to the neurorehabilitation unit, she was alert and orientated with a marked non-fluent aphasia and moderate comprehension difficulties. She had severe word finding difficulties, with frequent semantic substitution errors and difficulty following complex commands, and reduced comprehension of low frequency words. She was able to read but this was slow. Her mood was noted to be low and she was tearful. She had right homonymous hemianopia and a third nerve palsy with partial ptosis and dilated pupil on the left. There was facial asymmetry consistent with a right upper motor neuron lesion. She had increased tone in the right arm and leg with reduced passive range of movements of the fingers of the right hand and of the right ankle. There was limitation of abduction of the right shoulder due to pain with mild subluxation of the joint. Power was reduced in the right upper limb (MRC grade 1–2) and in the right lower limb (grade 2–3). Sensation was reduced on the right side and the tendon reflexes were increased with an extensor plantar response on the right. There was increased tone throughout the right side with spasticity (Ashworth scale 1–2).

Investigations

Blood tests were all normal, including FBC, renal, liver profile, TFT, ESR, CRP, fasting lipid profile, Magnesium, Calcium, folate, vitamin B12, thrombophilia screen, homocysteine and methylmalonic acid. A standard 12 lead ECG was normal. The initial CT revealed a large intraparenchymal haematoma centred on the left temporal lobe (Fig. 29.1). CT Angiography showed no vascular abnormality. Subsequently a four vessel angiogram was also normal. After she deteriorated on day 3 an MRI was performed which revealed a large left MCA territory infarct with restricted diffusion within the whole of the left MCA territory, in addition to the existing haematoma (Fig. 29.2a, b).

Clinical Progress

A diagnosis was made of pre-eclampsia leading to left temporal intracerebral haemorrhage and subsequent left MCA territory infarction. As a result she presented with a dominant MCA syndrome, with aphasia, right sided hemiparesis, hemisensory loss and right homonymous hemianopia with an additional third nerve lesion. The patient was initially treated in the local stroke unit and transferred to the neurorehabilitation unit 50 days after the onset of her symptoms. She completed a 16-week course of intensive inpatient neurorehabilitation and made significant gains in mobility, communication and activities of daily living. Her comprehension improved

Fig. 29.1 Admission CT head (unenhanced axial image) 5 mm slice. There is a large acute intra-parenchymal haematoma centred on the left temporal lobe with surrounding oedema and localised mass effect. Blood products extend into the basal cisterns and there is a shallow left temporoparietal convexity subdural collection

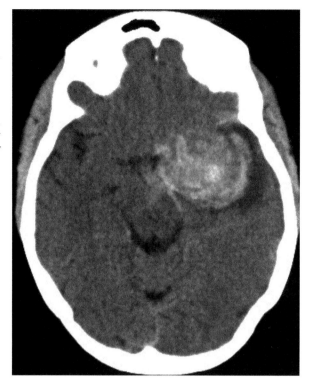

significantly such that she could follow and take part in conversations with support. She could mobilise with use of a walking stick and a rigid orthosis. She required a wheelchair for longer distances and outdoor mobility because of fatigue. She became independent for all personal care and some domestic tasks, including caring for her children. However, she had limited functional improvement in her right upper limb and developed spasticity, which was managed using a stretching and splinting regime and oral anti-spasticity agents (baclofen 20 mg tds and gabapentin 500 mg daily). She was discharged home at the end of the 16-week in-patient stay to the local integrated care team to continue rehabilitation in the community.

She was reviewed 4 months after discharge because of increasing spasticity affecting the right side. She had been discharged from the community team and found it difficult to implement her daily stretching and splinting programme by herself. The spasticity in her upper limb made it difficult for her to look after herself and dress independently and she had a marked associated reaction in the right arm when walking, which affected her balance. She attributed fatigue to the oral spasticity medications and was keen to reduce these. She continued to use an ankle foot orthosis (AFO) and now mobilised with one stick both indoors and outdoors. Her arm was held in a flexed position with flexion at the elbow, wrist and fingers (Fig. 29.3a, b). Tone was increased throughout the limb (Ashworth scale [1] ~ 2) (Table 29.1). Her spasticity was treated with botulinum toxin injection of biceps,

Fig. 29.2 MRI brain
performed 4 days after initial
presentation. (**a**) T2 axial
image; (**b**) Diffusion
weighted image (B1000). A
left temporal haematoma lobe
is hypointense on T2
weighted imaging consistent
with the recent bleed. There
is evidence of restricted
diffusion within the whole of
the left MCA territory in
keeping with an acute
infarct (**b**)

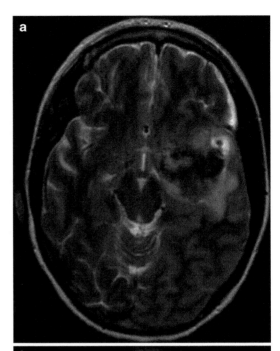

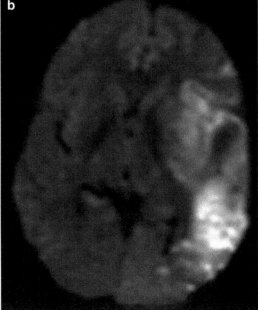

Fig. 29.3 (**a**, **b**) Pre botulinum toxin hand position

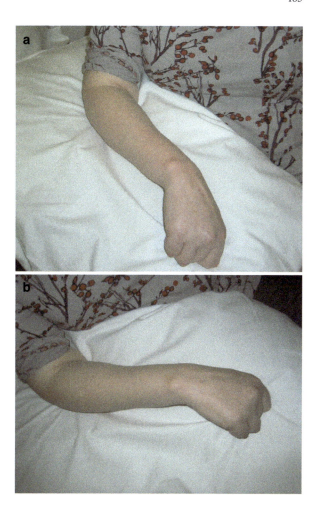

flexor carpi ulnaris, flexor carpi radialis, flexor digitorum superficialis and the lumbricals under EMG guidance. The goal of treatment was to facilitate the wearing of a splint, easier splint application and facilitation of a stretching programme.

The community physiotherapy team reviewed the response to treatment at the time of expected peak effect. Improvement in resting position and underlying spasticity was noted and goals were achieved (Fig. 29.4a, b). Four months later, spasticity re-emerged, requiring repeated assessment and botulinum toxin injection. Over the following 2 years, the patient was reviewed regularly in the focal spasticity clinic with repeated injections to muscles in the right upper limb, review of splinting and exercise regime to maintain the range in the arm and reduce troublesome

Table 29.1 Sequential outcome measures in response to treatment with botulinum toxin

Date Month/year	Ashworth (shoulder, elbow, wrist and hand)	Elbow Resting position (°flxn)/passive extension off neutral	Wrist Resting position (°flxn)/passive extension off neutral	MCPs Resting position (°flxn)/passive extension off neutral	PIPs Resting position (°flxn)/passive extension off neutral	ArMA (Max 24)	Muscles injected or review
01/11	2–3	100/0	35/15	80/0	100/0	16	Biceps, FCR, FCR, FDS, Lumbricals
05/11	0–1 pectorals 3	80/0	20/0	70/0	60/0 (wrist neutral)	10	Pectoralis major
11/11	2	65/0	20/0	70/0	90/0 (wrist flxd 45°)	15	FCR, FCU, FDS, lumbricals
03/12	2	70/0	40/25	70/0	100/0 (wrist flxd 40°)	10	FCR, FCU, FDS, FPL
07/12	2	90/0	30/15	80/0	100/0 (wrist flxd 40°)	15	Biceps, brachioradialis, FCR, FCU, FDS
08/12	0	70/0	10/0	40/0	50/0 (wrist neutral)	8	Review of effect of botulinum toxin
12/12	1–2	50/0	30/0	70/0	90/0 (wrist flxd 5°)	12	Biceps, brachioradialis, FCR, FCU, FDS
02/13	0	60/10	20/	40/0	0/0 (wrist neutral)	7	Review of outcomes

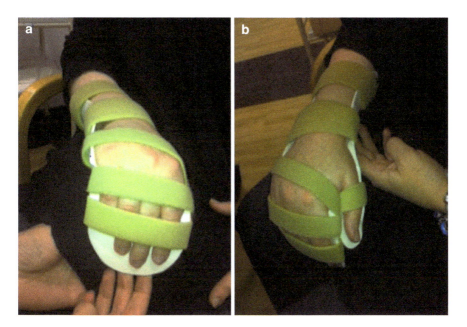

Fig. 29.4 (**a, b**) Post botulinum toxin hand position in splint

spasticity. Agreed goals of the botulinum toxin injections included relaxing the right hand and arm and to enabling better implementation of the splinting and stretching programme. Additional aims were to increase duration of wearing the splint and to improve the comfort and the resting position in the splint. Therapy interventions included progression of stretching and positioning programmes and splinting programmes as appropriate at 2 weeks after botulinum toxin injection and up to week 8 following each set of injections. The patient also worked on posture and core stability strengthening. Postural sets were progressed from crook lying into two point kneeling and standing. Over the following years gains were made in resting position, range and tone (Table 29.1). Using the Arm Activity Measure, section A for passive function (ARM-A) [2] the patient reported increased ease of care of her upper limb (score reduced from 16 out of a maximum of 24, to 7).

Discussion

This 38-year-old woman experienced an intracerebral haemorrhage and subsequent large MCA territory infarct as a consequence of pre-eclampsia 24 hours after the delivery of her baby by caesarean section. She had a significant dominant hemisphere syndrome with global aphasia, cognitive impairment, right sided facial weakness, visual field deficit, hemiparesis and hemisensory loss, the arm being more severely affected than her leg. No other underlying cause for her stroke was found. After a 4-month period of intensive specialist neurological rehabilitation she made considerable gains in function and independence. She required a further 6 months of rehabilitation in the community and thereafter, on-going speech and language therapy and spasticity management. The outcome measures shown in Table 29.1 track her response to botulinum toxin treatment and demonstrate the overall trend over time with an improvement in spasticity, resting posture, range of movement and ease of passive care as reflected in the ARM-A.

Spasticity can be a serious and activity-limiting consequence of stroke. Spasticity is defined as a velocity dependent increase in tonic stretch reflexes and is one component of the upper motor neurone syndrome. Spasticity occurring with motor dysfunction is common and is estimated to affect 38% of stroke survivors [3]. It is important that spasticity should be evaluated in the context of function, passive care and the presence of other neurological dysfunction. Untreated, spasticity can lead to increased loss of function, loss of range of movement at joints and muscle thixotrophy. In severe cases, contracture can develop and lead to maceration and breakdown of skin. All of these may lead to patient distress, poor function and reduced quality of life with increased burden of care and rehabilitation needs [4, 5]. Successful treatment has been shown to improve physical functioning and prevent secondary complications [6].

Upper limb spasticity after stroke is readily recognised clinically, but studies of the prevalence of the condition are lacking. One large prospective cohort study ($n = 106$) found that 31% of patients had upper limb spasticity at 12 months [3]. A more recent study ($n = 95$) found that 20% of stroke patients had upper limb spasticity 5 days after stroke and 18% had upper limb spasticity at 3 months [7]. Spasticity which emerges some months or even years after the onset of stroke highlights that increased tone after stroke is not a stable condition, but a dynamic one that needs to be addressed if causing problems. Despite the lack of prevalence or prospective cohort studies, upper limb spasticity after stroke is an important clinical issue and identification and treatment of spasticity is a key component of stroke rehabilitation.

The mainstay of treatment of spasticity involves physical measures, including mobilisation, using and stretching the limb, and a positioning and splinting programme. Any triggers of spasticity such as ill-fitting splints, infection or broken skin should also be identified and treated. Spasticity is amenable to pharmacological interventions because it is mediated by over-excitable stretch reflexes and loss of descending inhibitory control. Agents that act on or interact with the GABA system have been shown to be effective in treating spasticity and include baclofen, benzodiazepines, gabapentin, pregabalin and tizanidine. Agents which act directly on the muscle itself may also be useful e.g. dantrolene [8]. All these agents have a systemic effect and are particularly useful in people with widespread spasticity. At higher doses side effects may limit their use in people with stroke, who may be particularly susceptible to side effects of fatigue and cognitive slowing.

The advantage of botulinum toxin as a treatment for spasticity is that it can be administered directly into muscles affected by spasticity, avoiding the systemic side effects of orally administered drugs. Botulinum toxin is highly effective in reducing focal spasticity when administered in controlled doses to limited numbers of muscles and acts as a powerful neurotoxin on the presynaptic membrane, inhibiting the release of acetylcholine into the synaptic cleft and thus resulting in muscle weakness. The use of EMG to guide injections allows the presence of spasticity to be confirmed and ensures that injection is made into the appropriate muscle. The clinical effect of botulinum toxin begins within 7–14 days of injection and peaks at 3–6 weeks. The effect lasts 3–4 months; recovery is due to axonal sprouting. The period of muscle weakness can provide a "window of opportunity" to intensify physical measures and in which permanent changes can be made. There are many studies showing benefit in improving passive care, but there are conflicting results regarding recovery of function [9–11].

Measurement of spasticity and thus evaluation of the outcome of an intervention is crucial and in clinical practice the Ashworth scale is frequently used [1]. The resting position and range of movement around each joint as well as power should also be monitored. Patient reported measures are also useful and thus recording outcomes such as a numeric rating score (NRS: 0–10) can be helpful. In people with upper limb impairment the arm activity measure (Arm A and B) is a validated patient reported outcome measure, which can evaluate both active and passive function [2]. Over time, gains can be made, as this patient demonstrated, in whom the need for oral treatment was reduced improving her fatigue. The frequency and dose of botulinum toxin injection treatment can also be reduced over time in many patients because of the induction of permanent changes in the muscles. However, the dose of botulinum toxin that can be safely used is limited by the risks of systemic absorption and therefore it cannot be used to treat large numbers of muscles.

This case serves to highlight the benefit of co-ordinated multidisciplinary neuro-rehabilitation and effective spasticity management, allowing the patient to return to the highest possible level of function and independence, and preventing some of the long-term complications of stroke.

Key Clinical Learning Points
- Pre-eclampsia carries a significant vascular risk and can have devastating consequences
- People with stroke, particularly the young may have significant on-going rehabilitation needs that should be addressed to avoid long-term complications
- Post-stroke spasticity is a dynamic process which should be managed with a multidisciplinary approach combining physical and pharmacological intervention
- Botulinum toxin injections are a useful first-line pharmacological agent
- Outcome measures are an essential tool in monitoring treatment response to guide further management

References

1. Ashworth B. Preliminary trial of carisprodal in multiple sclerosis. Practitioner. 1964;192: 540–2.
2. Ashford S, Slade M, Turner-Stokes L. Conceptualisation and development of the arm activity measure (ArmA) for assessment of activity in the hemiparetic arm. Disabil Rehabil. 2013;35(18):1513–8.
3. Watkins CL, Leathley MJ, Gregson JM, et al. Prevalence of spasticity post stroke. Clin Rehabil. 2002;16(5):515–22.
4. Bhakta BB, Cozens JA, Chamberlain MA, et al. Impact of botulinum toxin type A on disability and carer burden due to arm spasticity after stroke: a randomised double blind placebo controlled trial. J Neurol Neurosurg Psychiatry. 2000;69(2):217–21.
5. Esquenazi A. Improvements in healthcare and cost benefits associated with botulinum toxin treatment of spasticity and muscle overactivity. Eur J Neurol. 2006;13 Suppl 4:27–34.
6. McCrory P, Turner-Stokes L, Baguley IJ, et al. Botulinum toxin A for treatment of upper limb spasticity following stroke: a multi-centre randomized placebo-controlled study of the effects on quality of life and other person-centred outcomes. J Rehabil Med. 2009;41(7):536–44.
7. Sommerfeld DK, Gripenstedt U, Welmer AK. Spasticity after stroke: an overview of prevalence, test instruments, and treatments. Am J Phys Med Rehabil. 2012;91(9):814–20.
8. Shakespeare DT, Boggild M, Young C. Anti-spasticity agents for multiple sclerosis. Cochrane Database Syst Rev. 2003;(4):CD001332.
9. Shaw LC, Price CI, van Wijck FM, et al. Botulinum Toxin for the Upper Limb after Stroke (BoTULS) Trial: effect on impairment, activity limitation, and pain. Stroke. 2011;42(5): 1371–9.
10. Cardoso E, Pedreira G, Prazeres A, et al. Does botulinum toxin improve the function of the patient with spasticity after stroke? Arq Neuropsiquiatr. 2007;65(3A):592–5.
11. Rousseaux M, Kozlowski O, Froger J. Efficacy of botulinum toxin A in upper limb function of hemiplegic patients. J Neurol. 2002;249(1):76–84.

Chapter 30
A Diagnosis Not to Forget

Sumanjit K. Gill

Clinical History

A 56-year-old lady presented to the rapid access TIA clinic via her GP after what she described as a 'funny turn' on the previous day. She was accompanied by her husband who gave the account of events. He described that she had walked into the kitchen and picked up some bread, asking him what he was doing with it. The ensuing conversation was punctuated by her repeatedly asking questions about the situation at the time of the turn e.g. how certain objects had come to be there and what they were doing in the kitchen. She recognised her husband and called him by his name. She had no problem walking or co-ordinating movements. He quickly realised that she was disorientated and called the doctor for an appointment. The whole event lasted a total of 30 min with a rapid and complete resolution. She had no past medical history of note.

Examination

When she was seen in the clinic, she had no clear recollection of the turn the previous day but could clearly recall events prior to, and after the event. On cognitive examination, she was completely orientated and scored full marks on the Montreal Cognitive Assessment Test. Physical and neurological examination was normal apart from a raised blood pressure of 156/70.

S.K. Gill, BSc Hons, MBBS, MRCP
Education Unit, National Hospital for Neurology and Neurosurgery,
UCL Institute of Neurology, London, UK
e-mail: sumanjit.gill@nhs.net

© Springer-Verlag London 2015
S.K. Gill et al. (eds.), *Stroke Medicine: Case Studies from Queen Square*,
DOI 10.1007/978-1-4471-6705-1_30

Investigations and Clinical Progress

An ECG showed left ventricular hypertrophy. MRI brain (Fig. 30.1) showed leuko-araiosis with prominent perivascular spaces. A diagnosis was made of an episode of transient global amnesia. Hypertension was also diagnosed as an independent finding and was treated with standard antihypertensive medication.

Discussion

The term transient global amnesia (TGA) was first used by Fisher and Adams after the clinical features were described by Guyotat and Courjon in 1956 [1, 2]. Prior to this the terms 'amnesic spells' or 'ictus amnésique' were used. TGA is characterised by the sudden onset of anterograde amnesia and is characterised by perseveration and repetitive questioning. There are several reported triggers for the attacks, including extremes of temperature, immersion in cold water, travel to unfamiliar places, emotional or painful events, a Valsalva manoeuvre, and exercise, including coitus. The duration of the majority of attacks is between

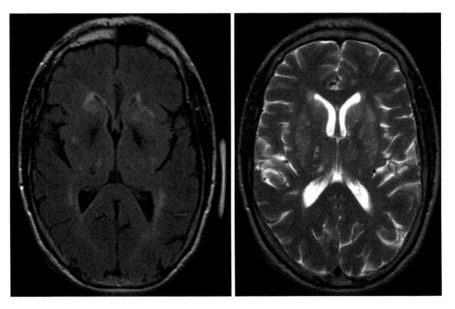

Fig. 30.1 Axial MR images FLAIR (*left*) and T2 weighted (*right*) sequences showing bilateral lesions in the white and deep grey structures in keeping with small vessel disease, and some prominent perivascular spaces

2 and 8 hours. The symptoms usually completely resolve with no residual symptoms of memory impairment other than for the event or the 1 or 2 hours preceding it. Occasionally, detailed neuropsychological testing may show mild long-term impairment of memory but whether such findings are related to the episode of TGA is uncertain.

TGA is a condition seen more commonly in older patients, usually over the age of 50. The incidence is 23.5–32 per 100,000 per year [3]. Patients can be reassured that recurrence is unusual, although about 5% of patients will experience a recurrence.

The aetiology of TGA remains unclear. The differential diagnosis includes TIA, epilepsy and migraine but in such cases there are usually other features during the attack to suggest the alternative diagnosis. It is clear that TGA is distinct from TIA and is not itself an indicator of cerebrovascular disease, because follow up studies show no increase in the risk of future stroke compared to matched controls [4]. TGA can be accompanied by headache and nausea and there is an association with a prior history of migraine, suggesting that cortical spreading depression may have a role to play [5]. The main differential diagnosis is transient epileptic amnesia (TEA), which has several clinical features to distinguish it from TGA. Most notably, personal identity is lost in TEA and not in TGA. Epileptic attacks tend to occur more frequently and have a shorter duration. They also occur on waking which is not a characteristic of TGA [6].

Diagnostic criteria were first clearly described by Hodges and Warlow in 1990 [7]. These are given in Box 30.1 below.

> **Box 30.1 Diagnostic Criteria for Transient Global Amnesia**
> 1. The sudden onset of inability to recall new information
> 2. Preservation of personal identity
> 3. A witness account of events
> 4. No focal neurological signs
> 5. Complete resolution within 24 hours except for amnesia for the event and the hours preceding it

Imaging studies using diffusion weighted scanning have reported either normal findings or in small percentage of cases, hippocampal changes [8, 9]. Rarely, imaging will show an underlying temporal lobe glioma. Rather than lending weight to a particular aetiology for TGA, the finding of alternate pathology in a number of cases on imaging should encourages us to keep our minds open to a differential diagnosis when faced with these cases. The finding of enlarged perivascular spaces (or Virchow Robin spaces) as seen in this case is a feature of the ageing brain and is associated with hypertension and small vessel disease. It has been demonstrated in one study of 97 males that an increased number of enlarged perivascular spaces is associated with mildly impaired cognitive function [10]. There is no known association with transient global amnesia.

Key Clinical Learning Points
1. Transient global amnesia has been shown not to have a vascular aetiology
2. Despite this, it is usually an event experienced by the older population and usually seen in those over the age of 50
3. It has various triggers including emotional stress and extremes of temperature
4. The main differential diagnosis is transient epileptic amnesia
5. It is not usually associated with persistent cognitive impairment

References

1. Fisher CM, Adams RD. Transient global amnesia. Acta Neurol Scand. 1964;40(9):1–83.
2. Pearce JMS, Bogousslavsky J. Les ictus amnesiques and transient global amnesia. Eur Neurol. 2009;62:188–92.
3. Koski KJ, Marttila RJ. Transient global amnesia: incidence in an urban population. Acta Neurol Scand. 1990;81:358–60.
4. Hodges JR, Warlow CP. The aetiology of transient global amnesia. Brain. 1990;113:639–57.
5. Zorzon M, Antonitti L, Mase G, et al. Transient global amnesia and transient ischaemic attack. Stroke. 1995;26:1536–42.
6. Owen D, Paranandi B, Sivakumar R, et al. Classical diseases revisited: transient global amnesia. Postgrad Med J. 2007;83(978):236–9.
7. Hodges JR, Warlow CP. Syndromes of transient amnesia: towards a classification. A study of 153 cases. J Neurol Neurosurg Psychiatry. 1990;53(10):834–43.
8. Huber R, Aschoff AJ, Ludolph AC, et al. Transient global amnesia: evidence against vascular ischaemic aetiology from diffusion weighted imaging. J Neurol. 2002;249:1520–4.
9. Ahn S, Kim W, Lee Y-S, et al. Transient global amnesia: seven years of experience with diffusion-weighted imaging in an emergency department. Eur Neurol. 2011;65:123–8.
10. MacLullich AMJ, Wardlaw JM, Ferguson KJ, et al. Enlarged perivascular spaces are associated with cognitive function in healthy men. J Neurol Neurosurg Psychiatry. 2004;75:1519–23.

Chapter 31
A Migraine with Persistent Focal Symptoms

David Bradley and Robert Simister

Clinical History

A 38-year-old right-handed sales assistant presented to the emergency department complaining of severe right side throbbing headache associated with nausea, movement sensitivity and photophobia. The headache began while bathing her children and it was preceded by a brief episode of visual blurring, followed by tingling and numbness starting in the right hand and spreading to the right hand side of her face and also her leg.

She had a background history of regular similar migraine headaches, which were accompanied by a visual aura in about half the attacks. However, she had not previously experienced sensory symptoms. She was known to have sickle cell trait and was not on any regular medications.

An initial clinical diagnosis of migraine with aura was made. However, the next morning her sensory symptoms were still present.

Examination

The patient was alert and orientated. General examination and routine observations were normal. Cranial nerve examination revealed subjective reduced sensation in a patchy distribution on the right side of the face. Limb examination showed normal

D. Bradley, MRCPI, PhD
Stroke and Acute Brain Injury Unit, National Hospital for Neurology and Neurosurgery, London, UK
e-mail: davidbradley@physicians.ie

R. Simister, MA, FRCP, PhD (✉)
Comprehensive Stroke Service, National Hospital for Neurology and Neurosurgery, UCLH Trust, London, UK
e-mail: robert.simister@nhs.net

© Springer-Verlag London 2015
S.K. Gill et al. (eds.), *Stroke Medicine: Case Studies from Queen Square*,
DOI 10.1007/978-1-4471-6705-1_31

tone, power, co-ordination and reflexes. Sensory examination showed loss of light touch and pain sensation in a patchy distribution throughout the right side of the body.

Investigations

Routine bloods and ECG were normal. An urgent CT, carried out to rule out haemorrhage, was normal. MRI brain showed restricted diffusion consistent with acute infarction in the left PCA territory, involving the left thalamus, lingual gyrus and the splenium of the corpus callosum (Fig. 31.1 and 31.2). Stroke workup was completed with a normal echocardiogram, thrombophilia screen and vascular imaging.

Her symptoms were attributed to a diagnosis of cerebral infarction in the left PCA territory secondary to migraine.

Discussion

An association between migraine and stroke has been recognised for many years, although the role of migraine as an independent vascular risk factor for stroke in the population remains controversial [1]. Several large meta-analyses indicate that patients with migraine have an approximately two-fold increased frequency of stroke, and that *migraine with aura* (which represents approximately one third of migraineurs [2]) is the group in which the main effect is seen [3–5]. These analyses indicate that the association is particularly marked in young women, and it has further been suggested that that smoking and the use of estrogen containing oral contraceptive medication enhances the risk in patients with migraine by as much as 10-fold [6].

Several disorders are characterised by both episodic migraine and stroke (or stroke-like episodes), for example Cerebral autosomal-dominant arteriopathy with stroke-like episodes and leukoencephalopathy (CADASIL) [7], mitochondrial disorders, including the syndrome of mitochondrial encephalopathy, lactic acidosis, and stroke-like episodes (MELAS) [8], the anti-phospholipid antibody syndrome and systemic lupus erythematosis [9]. The combination of a positive family history for both migraine and stroke should lead to genetic screening for these disorders in younger patients with otherwise unexplained stroke.

More recently, there has also been interest (and significant controversy) in a possible bi-directional association between patent foramen ovale (PFO) and migraine [10] (i.e., that PFO may result in both stroke and migraine, and on the other hand that PFO may occur more frequently in migraineurs), although it is worth noting that the importance of PFO in stroke is itself debated. Whilst the presence of a

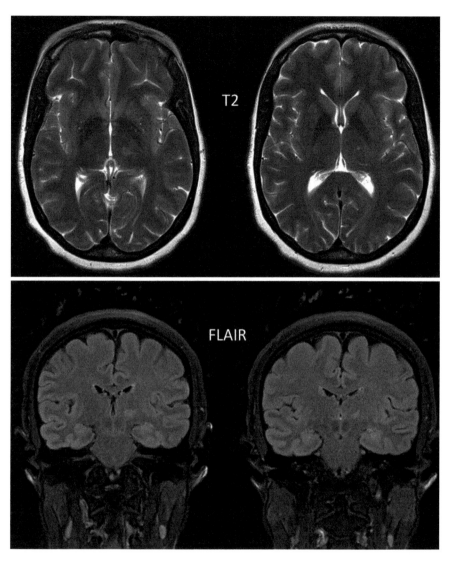

Fig. 31.1 Axial T2 (*top left*), and Coronal FLAIR (*bottom left*) sequences show acute ischaemic lesions in the left thalamus and left lingual gyrus. See also fig. 31.2 below

patent foramen ovale appears to be a risk factor for first stroke in younger patients [11], closure of a PFO in patients with cryptogenic stroke does not seem to reduce risk of stroke recurrence [12].

Migraine is categorised as a vascular headache syndrome. Possible mechanisms for ischaemic stroke in association with a migraine attack include both direct mechanisms e.g., vasoconstriction during a migraine aura leading to impaired flow and indirect mechanisms e.g. hypercoagulability, platelet activation or thrombosis as a result of slow flow during a migraine attack. However, studies of "migraineous infarction" are limited. The reduction in blood flow seen with spreading cortical depression is not thought to be in the ischaemic range, but it is possible that in rare cases the reduction in flow is sufficient to result in infarction. One issue to bear in mind, is that stroke in a migraineur may itself precipitate a migraine attack. This is particularly common in patients with carotid artery dissection and occlusion, and in most cases migraine in a patient in stroke is secondary to the stroke rather than causative [13]. Thus, our policy is only to diagnose migraineous infarction when the symptoms of stroke arise in a patient with established history of migraine, and evolve from an otherwise typical migraine aura, the infarction is in the typical territory of the migraine aura (i.e., typically PCA territory, as in this case) and no other cause is evident after extensive investigation.

There are a number of red flags that should prompt consideration and investigation for cerebral infarction when a patient presents with an apparent migraine associated with focal symptoms, as follows:

- Prolonged aura (greater than 1 hour).
- Negative symptoms e.g., dark scotoma or field loss rather than bright flashing lights (photopsia) or true numbness rather than pins & needles.
- Fixed, non-evolving features otherwise typical of migraine aura.
- Significant increase in aura frequency or significant change in aura type.
- First occurrence of migraine aura at an older age (e.g. >50 years).

Apart from showing infarction, usually small infarcts in the occipital lobe, there are no specific imaging characteristics of migraineous stroke. A number of reports describe an excess of white matter hyperintensities in migraineurs on MRI, but whether this is a causal relationship is uncertain, although they do not appear to be associated with standard vascular risk factors [14]. Attack frequency does seem relevant [15], and in keeping with the common site of migraineous infarction, the posterior circulation appears to be more at risk for the accumulation of white matter hyperintensities in migraine [16].

There does not appear to be any association between triptan use and stroke in migraineurs [17], but some experts probably inappropriately, recommend avoiding their use in patients with migraine with aura. There is no evidence to support the use of antiplatelets in patients with migraine with aura without another indication (i.e., established vascular disease). Smoking cessation and avoidance of the combined contraceptive pill are advocated. The mainstay of acute management of migraine with aura is non-steroidal anti-inflammatory drugs and standard preventive medications may be used, although beta-blockers may worsen migraine aura frequency [18].

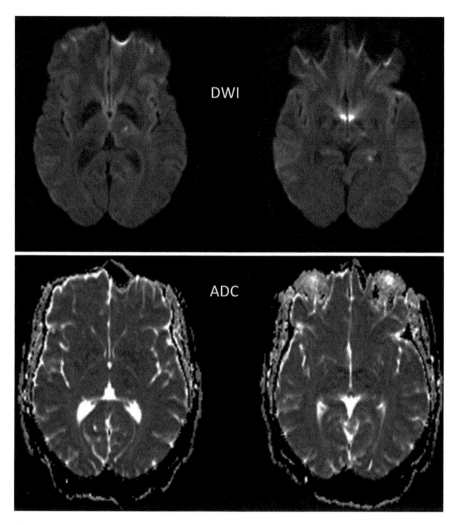

Fig. 31.2 Acute restricted diffusion consistent with acute infarction in the distribution of the left posterior cerebral artery on diffusion weighted (*upper images*) and ADC mapping (*lower images*)

Key Clinical Learning Points
1. Migraine with aura is associated epidemiologically with a two-fold increase in ischaemic stroke frequency, and the rate is higher in young women and with smoking and use of combined oral contraceptives; migraine without aura is not associated with increased stroke frequency
2. A direct causal relationship between stroke and migraine at the time of onset of the stroke should not be assumed and in many cases the migraineous symptoms will be secondary to the stroke, not vice versa

3. Migraineous infarction should only be diagnosed in a patient with an established history of migraine and when the symptoms of stroke evolve from an otherwise typical migraine aura, the infarction is in the typical territory of the migraine aura (i.e., typically occipital) and no other cause is evident after extensive investigation

4. Triptans and ergots, while not proven to be detrimental, are frequently avoided in patients with migraine aura due to the theoretical risk of worsening the reduced blood flow associated with cortical spreading depression. Triptans are contra-indicated in patients with established vascular disease

5. Migraine by itself should not be treated as a vascular risk factor with preventive medications. Similarly, migraineurs who develop stroke require full vascular workup for the causes of stroke and any vascular risk factors should managed in the usual way. In particular, smoking cessation and avoidance of oestrogenic contraceptive medication should be advocated

Key Radiological Learning Points

1. MR Imaging is an important investigation when infarction is suspected in a migraineur, to look for evidence of acute pathology (for example infarction or haemorrhage) and relevant underlying disease (for example CADASIL or MELAS)

2. Non-specific white matter hyperintensities on MRI are more commonly seen in migraineurs, and their nature and importance are not well understood. They do not by themselves represent an indication for secondary prevention medication

References

1. Bousser MG, Welch KM. Relation between migraine and stroke. Lancet Neurol. 2005;4:533–42.
2. Ferrari MD. Migraine. Lancet. 1998;351:1043–51.
3. Etminan M, Takkouche B, Isorna FC, et al. Risk of ischaemic stroke in people with migraine: systematic review and meta-analysis of observational studies. Br Med J. 2005;330:63.
4. Schurks M, Rist PM, Bigal ME, et al. Migraine and cardiovascular disease: systematic review and meta-analysis. Br Med J. 2009;339:b3914.
5. Spector JT, Kahn SR, Jones MR, et al. Migraine headache and ischemic stroke risk: an updated meta-analysis. Am J Med. 2010;123:612–24.
6. MacClellan LR, Giles W, Cole J, et al. Probable migraine with visual aura and risk of ischemic stroke: the stroke prevention in young women study. Stroke. 2007;38:2438–45.
7. Chabriat H, Joutel A, Dichgans M, et al. Cadasil. Lancet Neurol. 2009;8:643–53.
8. Pavlakis SG, Phillips PC, DiMauro S, et al. Mitochondrial myopathy, encephalopathy, lactic acidosis, and strokelike episodes: a distinctive clinical syndrome. Ann Neurol. 1984;16:481–8.
9. Tjensvoll AB, Harboe E, Goransson LG, et al. Migraine is frequent in patients with systemic lupus erythematosus: a case-control study. Cephalalgia. 2011;31:401–8.

10. Schwedt TJ, Demaerschalk BM, Dodick DW. Patent foramen ovale and migraine: a quantitative systematic review. Cephalalgia. 2008;28:531–40.

11. Overell JR, Bone I, Lees KR. Interatrial septal abnormalities and stroke: a meta-analysis of case-control studies. Neurology. 2000;55:1172–9.

12. Furlan AJ, Reisman M, Massaro J, et al. Closure or medical therapy for cryptogenic stroke with patent foramen ovale. N Engl J Med. 2012;366:991–9.

13. Olesen J, Friberg L, Olsen TS, et al. Ischaemia-induced (symptomatic) migraine attacks may be more frequent than migraine-induced ischaemic insults. Brain. 1993;116(Pt 1):187–202.

14. Swartz RH, Kern RZ. Migraine is associated with magnetic resonance imaging white matter abnormalities: a meta-analysis. Arch Neurol. 2004;61:1366–8.

15. Kruit MC, van Buchem MA, Hofman PA, et al. Migraine as a risk factor for subclinical brain lesions. JAMA. 2004;291:427–34.

16. Kruit MC, van Buchem MA, Launer LJ, et al. Migraine is associated with an increased risk of deep white matter lesions, subclinical posterior circulation infarcts and brain iron accumulation: the population-based MRI CAMERA study. Cephalalgia. 2010;30:129–36.

17. Hall GC, Brown MM, Mo J, et al. Triptans in migraine: the risks of stroke, cardiovascular disease and death in practice. Neurology 2004;62:563–8.

18. Hedman C, Andersen AR, Andersson PG, et al. Symptoms of classic migraine attacks: modifications brought about by metoprolol. Cephalalgia. 1988;8:279–84.

Chapter 32
Stroke and Systemic Disease

David Collas

Clinical History

A 70-year-old retired female civil servant developed a blister and ulcer on her left ring finger associated with cyanosis of the distal phalanges. There was some pain at the tips but no paraesthesiae. She had given up smoking 3 years ago, after 52 pack-years. Her past history included hypertension treated with amlodipine, bladder prolapse and fibroids. She had active rheumatoid arthritis and was being treated with prednisolone, methotrexate and salazopyrine.

Examination

After a week she consulted her GP who also noticed black spots on the tips of her middle and ring fingers, and recorded a marked difference in blood pressure between the two arms, being 180/110 on the right but only 100/80 mmHg on the left affected side. She was referred to a vascular surgeon.

More detailed examination revealed that both radial pulses were present but weaker on the left, and there was a complete absence of pulses below the femoral arteries, with discolouration of the third toe on the left foot, thought the rest of the foot was warm and well-perfused. The initial differential diagnosis of left subclavian stenosis was widened to include aortic thrombus, cardio-embolic events and vasculitis.

D. Collas, BSc, MB, BS FRCP
Stroke Medicine, Watford General Hospital, Watford, UK
e-mail: david.collas@nhs.net

© Springer-Verlag London 2015
S.K. Gill et al. (eds.), *Stroke Medicine: Case Studies from Queen Square*,
DOI 10.1007/978-1-4471-6705-1_32

Investigations and Subsequent Progress

She proceeded to CT angiography 15 days after her first symptoms. This showed significant atheroma of the aortic arch (Fig. 32.1) with soft plaque causing near occlusion of the left subclavian artery 3 cm from its origin , which was confirmed on catheter angiography (Fig. 32.2). The abdominal aorta had significant plaque with mixed plaque at the origin of the left iliac artery.

A vasculitic screen was carried out: ANA was positive at a titre of 1:100, ENAs negative, c-ANCA negative, p-ANCA negative. The ESR had fluctuated between 50 and 93 mmHr over the previous 3 months and the C reactive protein was 169 mg/l. An echocardiogram showed a normal left ventricle in structure and function with no significant valvular heart disease.

Fig. 32.1 Coronal reconstructed image from a thoracic CT arteriographic study showing a partly calcified atheromatous mural plaque (*arrow*) in the aortic arch in the region of the great vessel origins

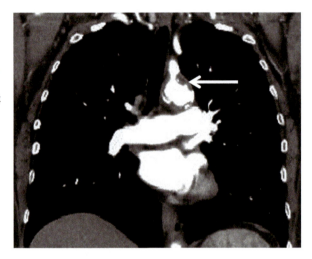

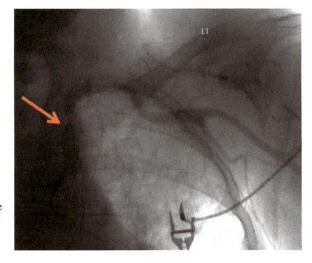

Fig. 32.2 Unsubtracted catheter angiographic image showing a filling defect in the left subclavian artery (*arrow*) resulting in near total occlusion

Clinical Progress

Initial management included an unfractionated heparin infusion followed by a prostacyclin infusion and subsequent subclavian angioplasty the following day. Three hours post procedure she was noticed to be pale, weak and sweating with a left face, arm and leg weakness. She also had left sided neglect. Her NIH Stroke Score was calculated at 13. She had a CT scan, which showed no early changes so she was considered a candidate for thrombolysis (Fig. 32.3a). Her heparin dose was minimal: 1,000 units given at the time of the angioplasty and therefore not a contraindication to thrombolysis, which was swiftly administered. The site of arterial puncture in the groin was observed for signs of bleeding but these were mild and easily managed with a pressure dressing.

Following thrombolysis her NIH Stroke Score fell to 6. The follow-up CT scan showed a moderate sized right frontal infarct (Fig. 32.3b).

Further blood tests to clarify the aetiology showed cholesterol 4 mmol/L, normal internal carotid arteries on duplex ultrasound with atheroma at the origin of the right external carotid artery, and fasting glucose 9.7 mmol/L. She remained in sinus rhythm on the cardiac monitor, later confirmed by 24-hour Holter monitor.

A rheumatologist was consulted and the diagnosis of rheumatoid vasculitis was made. She received pulsed methyl prednisolone for 3 days followed by oral prednisolone. The Ileoprost infusion was repeated daily for 1 week. A PET scan was performed to detect vasculitis elsewhere; and there was no evidence of

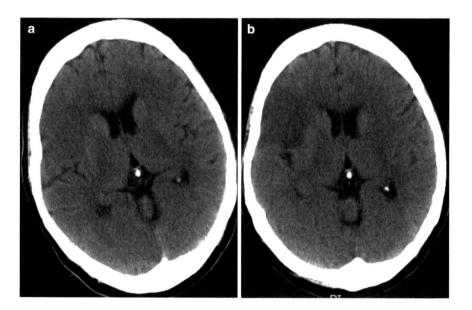

Fig. 32.3 Non contrast CT brain imaging (**a**) before and (**b**) 24 hours after thrombolysis showing subtle loss of grey white matter differentiation in the right frontal lobe which evolves to a more conspicuous infarct on subsequent study

inflammation within the walls of the aorta or great vessels, but there was increased activity around joints, particularly the hips and shoulders, in keeping with her known diagnosis of rheumatoid arthritis.

Occupational therapists assessment noted impulsivity, impaired planning and a lack of insight into her mild deficits. Her MOCA (Montreal Cognitive Assessment Score) was 24/30 with points lost on executive function, and language testing. She performed poorly at letter and number cancellation tests. By day 7 her weakness was limited to pronator drift of her left arm only. The lesions on her fingers were healing.

Discussion

Stroke is an uncommon complication of subclavian angioplasty. Thrombolysis in this situation is sometimes complicated by the pre-procedure use of heparin or in the case of emergency coronary angioplasty or stenting, high doses of antiplatelet drugs. There is uncertainty about the efficacy of intravenous alteplase in this situation as sometimes the embolus is composed of calcified plaque rather than thrombus, and also the possibility that the embolus is an air or device embolus. However, in one series of 66 patients where 18% of them were given thrombolysis (a combination of intravenous and intra-arterial treatment) a positive effect was demonstrated and no safety issues were identified [1].

Systemic vasculitis can have a variety of manifestations in the CNS, including stroke (either haemorrhage or infarct), seizures, anterior ischaemic optic neuropathy, and meningoencephalitis. Stroke can be due to an arterial occlusion secondary to inflammation of the blood vessel wall or due to a thrombotic angiopathy of the small blood vessels. Rheumatoid vasculitis rarely has any effect on the CNS and vasculitides causing stroke are more commonly seen in the setting of SLE, giant cell arteritis, and with Behcet's disease. Cerebral vasculitis has been described in severe cases of rheumatoid arthritis, usually those who are seropositive and a full systemic examination should be carried out when investigating a cryptogenic stroke to look for extraarticular manifestations of disease [2].

Key Clinical Learning Points
1. There is a risk of stroke from subclavian angioplasty and it is safe to consider thrombolysing these patients
2. The cause of stroke may often be multifactorial and in this case all possibilities should be considered and treated
3. Systemic vasculitis can be a cause of ischaemic stroke

References

1. Khatri P, Taylor R, Palumbo V, et al. The safety and efficacy of thrombolysis for strokes after cardiac catheterisation. J Am Coll Cardiol. 2008;51(9):906–11.
2. Akrout R, Bendjemaa S, Fourati H, et al. Cerebral rheumatoid vasculitis: a case report. J Med Case Reports. 2012;6:302.

Chapter 33
An Unusual Hypertensive Headache

Pervinder Bhogal

Clinical History

A 67-year-old retired cardiac theatre administrator with uncontrolled hypertension presented to the accident and emergency department with a 4-day history of acute onset left sided headache and blurred vision. The headache was severe and throbbing in character and associated with retro-orbital pain that varied in severity.

In addition to hypertension she had a past medical history of COPD and lower back pain. She was obese with a BMI of 45 and has a 60-pack year history of smoking.

Examination

She was alert, orientated and apyrexial. She was hypertensive with an initial blood pressure of 180/80. Her blood pressure periodically increased reaching a maximum of 260/140. She noticed that at the times of the increase in blood pressure her retro-orbital pain worsened. Examination of the central and peripheral nervous system was normal. She did not have any audible carotid bruits. Visual acuity was 6/6 bilaterally. There was no relative afferent pupillary defect. Heart sounds were normal with no added sounds.

P. Bhogal, MBBS, MRCS, FRCR, PG Dip MedEd
Atkinson Morley Department of Neuroradiology,
St. Georges Hospital, London, UK
e-mail: bhogalweb@aol.com

© Springer-Verlag London 2015
S.K. Gill et al. (eds.), *Stroke Medicine: Case Studies from Queen Square*,
DOI 10.1007/978-1-4471-6705-1_33

Investigations

Routine blood tests were normal and a 12 lead ECG showed sinus rhythm without ventricular hypertrophy. A plain CT head was normal, but CTA demonstrated a 3 mm left carotid-ophthalmic aneurysm.

Management

It was concluded that her headache, retro-orbital pain and visual symptoms were the result of the carotid-ophthalmic aneurysm. After multidisciplinary discussion with a surgeon and interventional neuroradiologist, it was decided to proceed to endovascular treatment of the aneurysm after informed consent. At preliminary carotid catheter angiography, it became evident that the left ophthalmic artery originated from the neck of the aneurysm (Fig. 33.1). In view of the risk that occluding the ophthalmic artery during coiling of the aneurysm would cause loss of vision, it was decided to perform a test occlusion of the artery. Therefore, with the patient awake, an intravascular balloon was inflated in the left internal carotid artery across the origin of the ophthalmic artery, preventing blood flowing from the internal carotid artery into the ophthalmic artery. Clinically the patient did not experience any visual loss and fundoscopy performed by a consultant ophthalmologist, repeated over 20 min, was normal with continued flow within the central retinal artery.

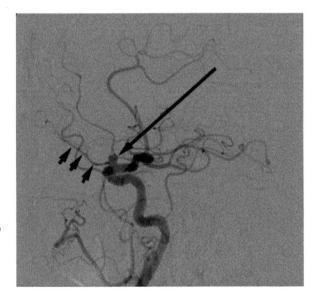

Fig. 33.1 A lateral image from an internal carotid angiogram demonstrates the aneurysm (*long black arrow*) and the ophthalmic artery (*short black arrows*) originating from the aneurysm neck

Fig. 33.2 Two coils were placed in the aneurysm resulting in successful exclusion of the aneurysm from the circulation (*long white arrow*). However, the ophthalmic artery was also occluded (*short white arrows* demonstrate the path of the previously identified ophthalmic artery)

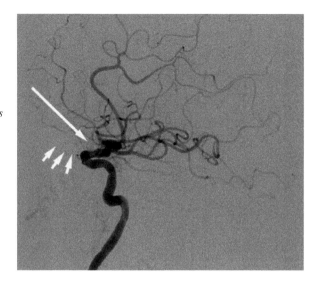

The neuroradiologist then proceeded to coil the aneurysm under general anaesthesia, occluding the aneurysm but also the ophthalmic artery (Fig. 33.2). She received 500 mg I.V. aspirin during the procedure and was commenced on oral aspirin (75 mg daily) as well as treatment dose low molecular weight heparin with the aim of preventing thrombosis within the ophthalmic artery. She awoke from the anaesthetic with no visual symptoms.

Her initial recovery was uneventful. However, on day 4 after the procedure while bending over, she suddenly developed a visual field defect in the left eye. Fundoscopy demonstrated emboli within the central retinal artery. After discussion with the stroke team and the ophthalmologists, the decision was made to treat her with ocular massage and acetazolamide. She made a complete recovery.

Discussion

The ophthalmic artery is typically the first major branch of the internal carotid artery and it enters the orbit via the optic canal, although other variants are well described. The central retinal artery is a major branch of the ophthalmic artery and it is responsible for supply to the inner retinal layers. Whilst the central retinal artery is essentially an end artery, there are normally anastomoses to the ophthalmic artery from branches of the external carotid artery. In the case described it is likely that these anastomoses maintained flow to the central retinal artery during the balloon occlusion. However, when the patient suffered an embolic event, presumably from thrombus at the site of occlusion of the ophthalmic artery at its origin, the central retinal artery became occluded leading to the episode of visual loss.

The main aim of the acute management of central retinal artery occlusion is to maintain perfusion pressure within the retinal circulation. This can be achieved in a variety of ways but can be broadly sub-divided into:

- Reducing intra-ocular pressure (IOP)
- Dilating the ophthalmic and central retinal arteries
- Increasing the ophthalmic artery pressure

Both ocular massage and intravenous acetazolamide reduce IOP and are probably the most widespread forms of treatment for central retinal artery occlusion in the acute setting [1]. An alternative method to reduce intra-ocular pressure is anterior chamber paracentesis although there is a lack of clinical efficacy for this technique[2].

Techniques to dilate the retinal arteries include ocular massage [1], inhalation of carbogen [3], and retrobulbar administration of vasodilators [1, 4]. The clinical benefit of the latter two techniques is doubtful and so they are not widely used [2].

Given the changes to both IOP and the vasodilator effect ocular massage has on the central retinal arteries, it has been postulated that this technique may cause mechanical disintegration of the clot. This was indeed seen in our case where it was noted that the clot fragmented and dispersed into the peripheral branches after ocular massage.

The limited success [5] and risk of intracerebral haemorrhage [6] associated with thrombolysis has resulted in the discontinuation of this treatment strategy.

Follow up of patients who have presented in either the acute or sub-acute stages of central retinal artery occlusion is essential, as is intensive treatment of vascular risk factors, because cardiovascular disease is the most common cause of death in patients that have suffered retinal artery occlusion [7, 8].

Key Clinical Learning Points
1. The central retinal artery is derived from the ophthalmic artery and is an end artery
2. Important anastomoses exist between the ophthalmic artery and the external carotid artery branches that can maintain perfusion to the central retinal artery in even of occlusion of the proximal ophthalmic artery
3. Ocular massage represents the most effective and easiest treatment option for acute central retinal artery occlusion
4. Lifestyle and systemic risk modification is essential in the long term given the association of central retinal arterial occlusion with generalised cardiovascular disease

References

1. Ffytche TJ. A rationalisation of treatment of central retinal artery occlusion. Trans Ophthalmol Soc UK. 1974;94:468–79.
2. Atebara NH, Brown GC, Carter J. et al. Efficacy of anterior chamber paracentesis and carbogen in treating acute nonarteritic central retinal artery occlusion. Ophthalmology. 1995;102:2029–35.
3. Tsacopoulos M, David NJ. The effect of arterial PCO2 on relative retinal blood flow in monkeys. Investig Ophthalmol Vis Sci. 1973;12:355–45.
4. Gombos GM. Retinal vascular occlusion and their treatment with low molecular weight dextran and vasodlators: report of six year's experience. Ann Ophthalmol. 1978;10:579–83.
5. Bertram B, Wolf S, Fisches H, et al. Thrombolytic treatment of retinal arterial occlusion with plasminogen activator. Klin Monbl Augenheilkd. 1991;198:295–300.
6. Barth H, Stein H, Fasse A, et al. Intracerebral haemorrhage after systemic thrombolysis in patients with occlusion of the central retinal artery. Report of two cases. Ophthalmologe. 1996;93:739–44.
7. Savino PJ, Glaser JS, Cassidy J. et al. Retinal stroke. Is the patient at risk. Arch Ophthalmol. 1973;95:1185–9.
8. Pfaffenbach DD, Hollenhorst RW. Morbidity and survivorship of patients with embolic cholesterol crystalisation in the ocular fundus. Am J Ophthalmol. 1973;75:66–72.

Chapter 34
Recurrent Thunderclap Headaches

Nicholas F. Brown and Martin M. Brown

Clinical History

A 22-year-old female right-handed investment banker presented with a 3-week history of recurrent thunderclap occipital headaches. The headaches were initially frontal and left sided, then right sided, and then became occipital. She described the headaches as "being hit from behind by a bat" and subsequently "pounding" with associated photophobia and hyperacusis. Each headache was precipitated by physical exertion at the gym. The headaches initially lasted approximately 30 min but in the week before presentation were lasting 9–10 hours. There were no relieving factors.

She had no past medical history and was not on any regular medications. There was no family history of note. She did not smoke or drink alcohol, and denied recreational drug use. She had recently started taking diphenhydramine sleeping tablets and unnamed Chinese herbal supplements.

Examination

She was alert and oriented. Blood pressure was 110/68 mmHg. Cardiac, respiratory, and abdominal examination was unremarkable. Neurological examination including fundoscopy was normal. There were no visible rashes.

N.F. Brown, MBBS, MA, MRCP
Department of Neurology, Royal Free Hospital, London, London, UK
e-mail: n.brown4@nhs.net

M.M. Brown, MA, MD, FRCP (✉)
Brain Repair & Rehabilitation, UCL Institute of Neurology, University College London,
The National Hospital for Neurology and Neurosurgery, London, UK
e-mail: martin.brown@ucl.ac.uk

© Springer-Verlag London 2015
S.K. Gill et al. (eds.), *Stroke Medicine: Case Studies from Queen Square*,
DOI 10.1007/978-1-4471-6705-1_34

Investigations

Routine blood tests including CRP and ESR were normal. ECG displayed sinus rhythm.

MRI Brain revealed normal brain parenchyma, however MR Angiogram of the intracranial arteries (Fig. 34.1) demonstrated a widespread irregular calibre with beading of multiple arterial segments of the circle of Willis bilaterally consistent with a vasculopathic process. These findings were confirmed on a four-vessel catheter angiogram (Fig. 34.1). CT Abdomen with contrast revealed normal extracranial blood vessels.

Vasculitis and thrombophilia screens were negative. Cerebrospinal fluid opening pressure at lumbar puncture was 14 cm. It was acellular with normal protein and glucose, culture and viral serology was negative.

She was diagnosed with cerebral vasoconstriction syndrome and commenced on oral nimodipine. She was discharged home and her headaches gradually subsided. Repeat MR Angiogram (Fig. 34.2) of the intracranial vessels 5 months post presentation revealed normal intracranial vessels, confirming the diagnosis of reversible cerebral vasoconstriction syndrome (RCVS). Nimodipine was gradually withdrawn, and she remains headache free.

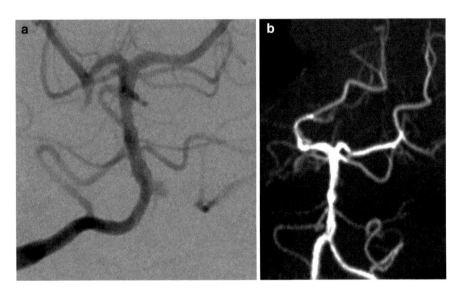

Fig. 34.1 (**a**) AP projection of right vertebral artery injection and (**b**) time of flight MR angiogram shows calibre irregularity of the basilar artery and subtle irregularity 'beading' of distal arterial segments (not shown)

Fig. 34.2 Interval MR angiogram 5 months post presentation. Normal intracranial vessels

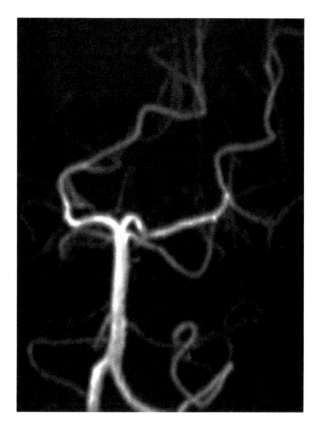

Discussion

Reversible cerebral vasoconstriction syndrome (RCVS) is characterised by transient dysregulation of cerebral vascular tone leading to prolonged but reversible constriction of intracranial arteries, with resolution within 3 months. Peak incidence is between 20 and 50 years of age, with a female predominance (2–10:1) [1, 2]. Accurate incidence is difficult to define as it is underdiagnosed, particularly in pure cephalgic cases.

The most common clinical presentation is with severe acute headache (typically thunderclap), with or without additional neurological symptoms including focal neurology (9–64%) and seizures (0–21%) [3–5]. The acute headache is typically bilateral, with posterior onset and associated nausea, vomiting, and photophobia. Most patients (>90%) will present with recurrent thunderclap headaches recurring 7 days apart on average, with a milder background headache between attacks [2, 5].

The pathophysiology of RCVS is not fully understood. Brain biopsies have not revealed abnormalities, and have not demonstrated vascular inflammation [6]. The prevailing hypothesis is that it is secondary to transient and reversible disturbance in the control of cerebral vascular tone, with subsequent multifocal and segmental arterial constriction and dilatation [4, 7]. Since intracranial vascular tone and calibre is dependent on both vascular receptor activity and sensitivity, a central vascular discharge (either spontaneous or evoked) with a multifactorial trigger may determine the relapsing and reversible nature of RCVS [3]. The temporal clinical progression suggests that the underlying disturbance first involves small distal arteries, potentially causing haemorrhage and a clinical syndrome identical to the posterior reversible encephalopathy syndrome, and then progresses to involve medium and large calibre vessels, with subsequent ischaemia and potential infarction [2].

The syndrome may be spontaneous (idiopathic), or may occur secondary to a precipitant (25–60%) [4]. Precipitants have been implicated from a temporal relationship with RCVS which may occur several months after precipitant use [3, 4]. Reported precipitants include vasoactive substances, pregnancy and the puerperium, catecholamine-secreting tumours, and immunosuppressants or blood products (Table 34.1). The most commonly reported precipitants are serotonin selective re-uptake inhibitors, cannabis, and over-the-counter nasal decongestants [2]. A trigger immediately prior to the onset of headache is recounted by 80% of patients, including sexual intercourse, straining, physical exertion, urination, high emotional state, showering, and head movements [4].

Complications of RCVS include seizures, PRES, subarachnoid haemorrhage, and intracerebral haemorrhage during the first 7 days after headache-onset when small calibre vessels are affected, followed by ischaemic infarcts during the second week when medium and larger calibre arteries are affected [4]. Subarachnoid haemorrhage is of small volume and tends to be localised, overlying the cortical surface with limited spread over 1–3 sulci [1, 4, 5]. Infarction is due to ischaemia distal to affected vessels, typically within arterial borderzone regions, and occurs in 7–50% of cases [1, 3–5].

CT/MR Brain imaging at presentation is frequently normal. Angiography, either transfemoral or indirect (MRA/CTA) shows multifocal segmental narrowing and dilatation, in a "string of beads" pattern. Typically the anterior and posterior cerebral circulations are bilaterally and diffusely affected, with potential involvement of the carotid artery and basilar siphon [4]. If performed in the first few days after presentation,

Table 34.1 Precipitants attributed to RCVS

Pregnancy and Puerperum
Vasoactive substances: Cocaine, Cannabis, Amphetamines, SSRIs, Nasal decongestants, ergotamine, methergine, bromocriptine, triptans, nicotine patches, ginseng
Catecholamine secreting tumours
Immunosuppressants or blood products: tacrolimus, cyclophosphamide, interferon-alpha, erythropoietin, intravenous immunoglobulin, packed red cells
Head trauma

Adapted from [4]

angiography may appear normal, due to the poor sensitivity of angiography to small vessel involvement. Follow-up cerebral imaging is abnormal in three quarters of cases, including infarcts (39%), subarachnoid haemorrhage (34%), intracerebral haemorrhage (20%), and oedema (20%) [5]. Serial angiography has found peak involvement of arterial segments 16 days after headache onset, with unsynchronised progression and regression of vasoconstricted arterial segments [1]. Complete reversal of angiographic abnormalities is apparent between 1 and 3 months after presentation.

Cerebrospinal fluid at presentation is frequently abnormal, and may show mild elevation in protein and white cell count [4]. Serum inflammatory markers may show a modest elevation [4].

The differential diagnosis for a single thunderclap headache includes primary headache syndromes, aneurysmal subarachnoid haemorrhage, intracranial haemorrhage, cervical or intracranial dissection, hypertensive encephalopathy, post-partum vasculopathy, venous thrombosis, giant cell arteritis, and pituitary apoplexy. Recurrent thunderclap headaches are much more likely to be RCVS or primary headache syndromes. Appropriate imaging and serum inflammatory markers should differentiate the above presentations. RCVS-SAH with vasospasm is distinguished from aneurysmal-SAH on imaging with typical appearances of a small volume bleed overlying the superior or lateral cortical surface, with multifocal vessel abnormalities remote from the site of bleeding, and no evidence of aneurysm rupture [1, 4, 5]. The differential diagnosis for the imaging appearances of RCVS is primary CNS angiitis but the clinical presentation of the two syndromes is very different. CNS angiitis rarely presents with thunderclap headache, progresses over more than 4 weeks, and has cerebrospinal fluid and serum abnormalities [6].

The following diagnostic criteria for RCVS have been proposed [3]:

1. Acute severe headache with or without neurological signs or symptoms
2. Multifocal segmental vasoconstriction of cerebral arteries demonstrated by angiography
3. No evidence for aneurysmal subarachnoid haemorrhage
4. Normal or near-normal cerebrospinal fluid analysis (protein <1 g/l, white cells <15 mm [4], glucose normal)
5. Reversibility of angiographic abnormalities within 12 weeks after onset

Initial management includes cessation of potential precipitants, blood pressure control, and medical management of seizures. There have been no clinical trials evaluating pharmacotherapy in RCVS and open studies have not found any significant clinical benefit with calcium channel blockers or glucocorticoids. Calcium channel blockers (particularly nimodipine) are frequently used as vasodilators, but care must be taken to avoid hypotension and subsequent borderzone infarction in areas perfused by the constricted artery [3, 5]. The optimum treatment duration is unclear. Patients with RCVS are sometimes given glucocorticoids at presentation due to diagnostic uncertainty of primary CNS angiitis and evidence of benefit in aneurysmal subarachnoid haemorrhage in animal studies [6]. However, there is no clear clinical indication for glucocorticoids in RCVS, and their use has been associated with a trend towards poor outcomes [5].

The prognosis in RCVS in favourable, with excellent recovery in uncomplicated cases. One series reported modified Rankin of 0–1 in 78% of patients, 2–3 in 11%, and 4–5 in 9% [5]. Cerebral infarction (but not haemorrhage) is associated with a poor outcome [5]. Deaths have rarely been reported. Relapse is very uncommon.

Key Clinical Learning Points
- RCVS is a transient disturbance in cerebral vascular tone with subsequent multifocal segmental intracerebral arterial constriction and dilatation
- RCVS should be considered in all presentations with cryptogenic strokes or thunderclap headache, particularly if recurrent
- Differentiation from primary CNS angiitis can be made clinically, and from aneurysmal subarachnoid haemorrhage radiologically
- Management includes enquiring about and discontinuing potential precipitants. Calcium channel blocker initiation may be beneficial
- Prognosis is favourable, but dependent on the extent of cerebral infarction

Key Radiological Learning Points
- All patients with recurrent thunderclap headaches with or without cerebral haemorrhage should have intracranial angiography
- Multifocal segmental narrowing and dilatation with a "string of beads" pattern on angiography (transfemoral or indirect), with normalisation within 3 months is diagnostic of RCVS
- Angiography at presentation may be normal, and repeat angiography may be required to demonstrate vascular abnormalities

References

1. Chen SP, Fuh JL, Wang SJ, et al. Magnetic resonance angiography in reversible cerebral vasoconstriction syndromes. Ann Neurol. 2010;67:648–56.
2. Ducros A, Boukobza M, Porcher R, et al. The clinical and radiological spectrum of reversible cerebral vasoconstriction syndrome. A prospective series of 67 patients. Brain. 2007;130:133–9.
3. Calabrese LH, Dodick DW, Schwedt TJ, et al. Narrative review: reversible cerebral vasoconstriction syndrome. Ann Intern Med. 2007;146:34–44.
4. Ducros A, Bousser MG. Reversible cerebral vasoconstriction syndrome. Pract Neurol. 2009;9:256–67.
5. Singhal AB, Hajj-Ali RA, Topcuoglu MA, et al. Reversible cerebral vasoconstriction syndromes. Analysis of 139 cases. Arch Neurol. 2011;68(8):1005–12.
6. Sattar A, Manousakis G, Jensen MB. Systematic review of reversible cerebral vasoconstriction syndrome. Expert Rev Cardiovasc Ther. 2010;8(10):1417–21.
7. Schwedt TJ, Matharu MS, Dodick DW. Thunderclap headache. Lancet Neurol. 2006;5:621–31.

Chapter 35
Stroke in Pregnancy

Ruth Law and Robert I. Luder

Clinical History

A 37-year-old, right-handed female who worked as a lecturer presented to the hyperacute stroke service with sudden onset right-sided weakness and aphasia. She was 36 weeks pregnant. Her husband described her as having stood up after breakfast and become suddenly unsteady and unable to speak. Her only past medical history was of migraine with visual aura but she had never experienced limb weakness or other neurological phenomena with migraine in the past. She took no medications. She had previously taken cocaine as a student but had used no recreational drugs for several years and was a non-smoker.

Examination

On examination she had a complete right hemiparesis and expressive dysphasia. Her NIHSS was 13. Her cardiovascular examination was normal with a blood pressure of 126/74 mmHg. Her heart rate was 92 beats per minute and an ECG showed sinus rhythm. The obstetric team were in attendance and a rapid foetal ultrasound scan revealed no acute obstetric issues. She was transferred for immediate brain CT and CTA.

R. Law, MA, MBBS, MRCP
Department of Medicine, University College London, London, UK
e-mail: Ruth.law2@nhs.net

R.I. Luder, BSc (Hons), FRCP (UK) (✉)
Department of Stroke Medicine, North Middlesex University Hospital,
Edmonton, London, UK
e-mail: robert.luder@nmh.nhs.uk

© Springer-Verlag London 2015
S.K. Gill et al. (eds.), *Stroke Medicine: Case Studies from Queen Square*,
DOI 10.1007/978-1-4471-6705-1_35

221

Investigations

CT brain showed changes consistent with an evolving left middle cerebral artery infarct and narrowing consistent with thrombus in the M1 segment on CTA (Figs. 35.1 and 35.2). She was transferred immediately to the angiography suite for endovascular intervention without receiving intravenous (IV) thrombolysis.

Fig. 35.1 Axial unenhanced CT image showing early ischaemic change in the left middle cerebral artery territory (*single white arrow*)

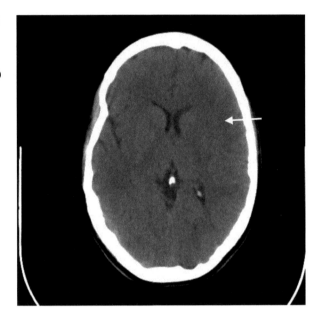

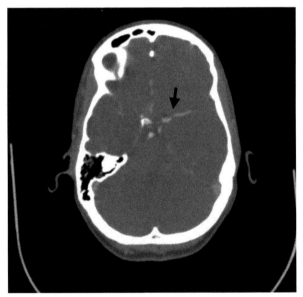

Fig. 35.2 Axial CT angiogram image showing narrowing of the left proximal middle cerebral artery (*black arrow*)

Catheter angiography demonstrated an unexpected right supra-clinoid carotid stenosis and near total occlusion of the left middle cerebral artery (MCA) correlating with the earlier CT findings. A Solitaire stent was selected to bridge the stenosis rather than attempting balloon expansion as there was a lower potential risk of fatal rupture. Following insertion of the stent a final angiogram demonstrated much-improved distal perfusion to the left hemisphere but around 60% residual stenosis. The total time from initial collapse at home to restoration of flow was under 4 hours.

The patient was transferred to the Intensive Care Unit for routine observation. On assessment the following day she had full power in her limbs and fluent speech. Some subtle naming difficulties with low frequency words remained.

An MRI DWI sequence that day demonstrated multiple small areas of restricted diffusion in keeping with acute infarcts (Fig. 35.3), predominantly affecting cortical areas in the left middle frontal gyrus, operculum and anterior aspect of insular cortex. She was discharged home after 72 hours on clopidogrel. A repeat MRI 2 months after the event revealed minimal parenchymal damage. She delivered a healthy baby boy 38 days post procedure insert full stop here.

Despite extensive further investigations including full thrombophilia and vasculitis screening, HIV testing, homocysteine levels, cardiac telemetry and Marfan's screening, the aetiology of the patient's stroke and her intracranial stenosis remained unclear. A bubble echocardiogram revealed a small patent foramen ovale but this was thought to be non-contributory. She was maintained on clopidogrel antiplatelet therapy and remained under regular review.

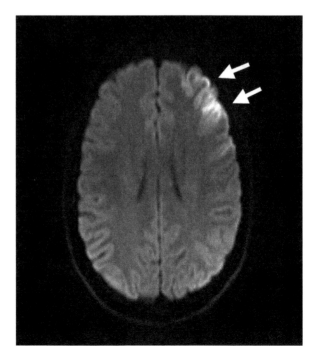

Fig. 35.3 Axial MRI B1000 DWI image showing relatively small area of cortical infarction in the left frontal lobe (*double white arrows*)

Discussion

Demographics

Published population figures vary widely in their estimate of stroke risk during pregnancy from 9 to 34 per 100,000 deliveries. This represents up to a threefold increased risk of stroke in pregnancy when compared with the normal population [1]. Haemorrhagic and ischaemic strokes are equally common [2]. There is also population based data to suggest that the incidence of stroke in pregnancy may be increasing [3]. Although there are rare pregnancy-specific causes of stroke such as amniotic fluid embolism, the commonest causes appear to be thrombophilia and cardioembolic disease [4].

Thrombolysis and endovascular thrombus extraction in Pregnancy

In this case the patient was not thrombolysed due to uncertainties at the time about its safe use in this context and because rapid intra-arterial intervention was available. According to the manufacturer's categorisation, the use of IV thrombolysis with tissue plasminogen activator (tPA) in pregnancy is relatively contraindicated. However there are many case reports in the literature of its safe and successful use in pregnancy by both the IV [5–7] and intra-arterial (IA) [8] route. Thrombolysis has also been used successfully in pregnancy for the treatment of pulmonary embolus and myocardial infarction. Endovascular thrombus extraction using a retrievable stent device is an option for treatment of stroke during pregnancy, either with or without prior intravenous thrombolysis. The risks of radiation exposure to the baby need to be considered, but this case demonstrates that feasibility of endovascular treatment in pregnancy. However, there are to date very few other case reports of the use of endovascular stenting for acute ischaemic stroke in pregnancy.

Key Clinical Learning Points
1. Pregnant women are at higher risk of stroke than the age matched general population
2. Published case series report that IV thrombolysis is safe for use in pregnancy in the treatment of acute ischaemic stroke
3. Our experience suggests that endovascular intervention is also a viable treatment option in certain cases
4. Pregnant women should be offered the same investigations and treatment as non-pregnant women

Key Radiological Learning Points
1. Immediate intracranial angiography is critical to demonstrating potentially treatable vascular lesions and is especially crucial if thrombolysis is contraindicated
2. MR/DWI can reveal the extent of infarction after stenting

References

1. Tate J, Bushnell C. Pregnancy and stroke risk in women. Womens Health. 2011;7(3):363–74.
2. Sharshar T, Lamy C, Mas JL. et al. Incidence and causes of strokes associated with pregnancy and puerperium. A study of public hospitals in Ile de France. Stroke. 1995;26:930–6.
3. Kuklina EV, Tong X, Bansil P, et al. Trends in pregnancy hospitalisations that included a stroke in the United States from 1994–2007. Reasons for concern? Stroke. 2011;42:2564–70.
4. Jaigobin C, Silver FL. Stroke and pregnancy. Stroke. 2000;31:2948–51.
5. Murugappan A, Coplin WM, Al-Sadat AN, et al. Thrombolytic therapy of acute ischaemic stroke during pregnancy. Neurology. 2006;66(5):768–70.
6. Leonhardt G, Gaul C, Nietsch HN, et al. Thrombolytic therapy in pregnancy. J Thromb Thrombolysis. 2006;21(3):271–6.
7. Wiese KM, Talkud A, Mathews M, et al. IV recombinant tPA in a pregnant woman with cardioembolic stroke. Stroke. 2006;37:2168–9.
8. Johnson DM, Kramer DC, Cohen E, et al. Thrombolytic therapy for acute stroke in late pregnancy with intra-arterial recombinant tPA. Stroke. 2005;36:e53–5.

Chapter 36
Cortical Blindness

Ruth Law and Robert I. Luder

Clinical History

A 73-year-old right-handed lady of Turkish origin presented to the hyperacute stroke unit with bilateral visual loss which had started the previous day. She had felt well until she went for her usual sleep in the afternoon. On waking around 14:00 she was unable to see anything, 'only black'. She experienced no headache or neck pain, no limb weakness and no change in speech. Distressed by her symptoms she lay in bed for a short while before telephoning her daughter for help.

She had a past medical history of a right lacunar stroke 5 years previously resulting in mild residual left sided weakness. She was a type 2 diabetic with a history of ischaemic heart disease and had undergone coronary artery bypass grafting 3 years previously. Her medications included aspirin, ramipril, furosemide, gliclazide and metformin. She lived alone, mobilised with a stick, was independent and has no reported cognitive problems.

Examination

On examination at presentation her blood pressure was 175/86 mmHg. Her heart rate was 60 and a 12-lead ECG revealed sinus rhythm. She had an ejection systolic murmur. There were no lateralising signs in the upper or lower limbs. On visual

R. Law, MA, MBBS, MRCP (✉)
Department of Medicine, University College London, London, UK
e-mail: Ruth.law2@nhs.net

R.I. Luder, BSc (Hons), FRCP (UK)
Department of Stroke Medicine, North Middlesex University Hospital,
Edmonton, London, UK
e-mail: robert.luder@nmh.nhs.uk

© Springer-Verlag London 2015
S.K. Gill et al. (eds.), *Stroke Medicine: Case Studies from Queen Square*,
DOI 10.1007/978-1-4471-6705-1_36

examination, acuity was markedly impaired – she was unable to differentiate light from dark. Her pupils were size 3 and reactive. Fundoscopy was unremarkable. She was unable to recognise movement in any part of her visual fields and did not startle to threat. Although she was unable to track an object, when instructed to move her eyes there was a full range of eye movements. The rest of the cranial nerve examination was normal.

Investigations

She was admitted to the hyperacute stroke service with a suspected diagnosis of cortical blindness. Her CT brain (Fig. 36.1) revealed bilateral wedge shaped low attenuation areas with loss of grey-white matter differentiation in the parieto-occipital lobes consistent with infarction in the posterior borderzones. CTA showed an irregular and very narrow right vertebral artery (Fig. 36.2), and a left vertebral artery compromised at its origin (Fig. 36.3). MRI with DWI (Fig. 36.4) supported these findings. Telemetry overnight showed several prolonged runs of broad complex tachycardia. She was reviewed urgently by the cardiology team who diagnose ventricular tachycardia and transferred her to the Intensive Care Unit where she was treated with bisoprolol, amiodarone and DC cardioversion. She reverted to a baseline rhythm of atrial fibrillation and remained stable. Her vision improved remarkably over the next few days, and she was transferred for ongoing rehabilitation 7 days after admission.

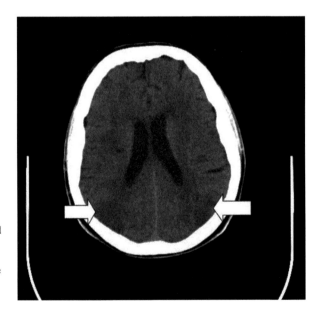

Fig. 36.1 Axial unenhanced CT showing bilateral areas of low density at parieto-occipital junctions indicative of infarction in the posterior borderzones

Fig. 36.2 CT angiography
showing irregular and
tortuous right vertebral
artery (*white arrows*)

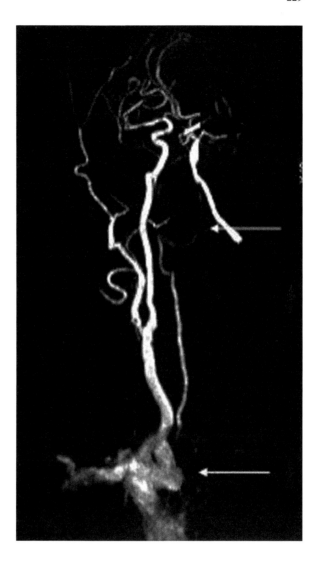

Fig. 36.3 CT angiography
showing kinked and
narrowed origin of left
vertebral artery (*white arrow*)

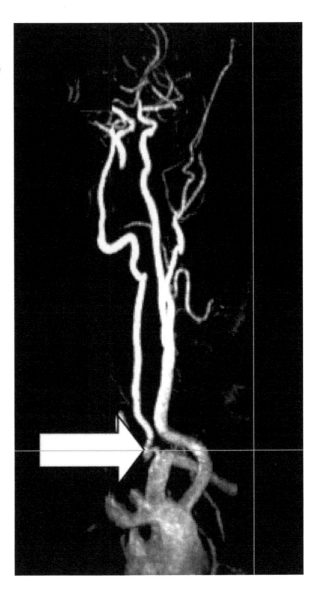

Fig. 36.4 B1000 Diffusion
weighted MRI sequence
showing bilateral areas
of acute infarction in
parieto-occipital junctions
(*white arrows*)

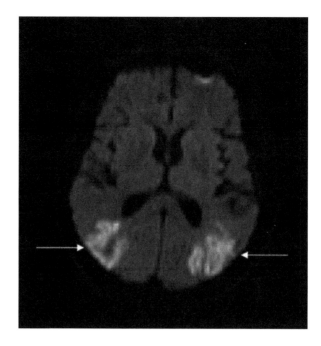

Discussion

Our patient developed simultaneous bilateral borderzone infarctions in the posterior borderzones between the PCA and MCA territories. affecting the visual cortex causing her syndrome of cortical blindness. This may have been associated with arrhythmia associated hypotension at some point associated with vertebral stenosis, which will have made her posterior circulation particularly vulnerable to border-zone infarction.

Cortical Blindness: Symptoms and Signs

Cortical blindness refers to a loss of vision secondary to bilateral dysfunction of the primary visual cortex or pathways. Our patient displayed the classical signs of complete cortical blindness; namely a loss of all visual sensation including light/dark appreciation and loss of visual response to threat, with intact pupillary responses, preserved extraocular movements and normal fundi.

Presentation varies according to how much of the optic pathway is affected. For example, it is thought that preservation of the extrageniculate pathway explains why some patients have preserved blink response to threat or can avoid objects despite apparent blindness on testing. Amnesia may also be a prominent feature if there is accompanying bilateral damage to the medial temporal lobes. With inferior temporal lobe involvement a restless, hyperactive state may accompany the loss of vision making assessment of the patient extremely challenging. Similar barriers to assessment arise in some cortically blind patients who display anosognosia (failure to recognise that they cannot see) compensating with confabulation, and denying visual impairment (Anton's Syndrome).

The diagnosis of cortical blindness is clinical, with the aid of neuroimaging to show anatomical correlation. CTA or MRA may provide useful information in relation to aetiology. The 12-lead ECG should also be reviewed and cardiac monitoring performed for at least 72 hours post presentation.

EEG is usually abnormal but not diagnostic, with slowing of the posterior dominant rhythm and absence of a well-developed alpha rhythm [1]. Visual evoked potentials are also non-contributory to diagnosis [1].

Any cerebral insult affecting the occipital lobes bilaterally can cause cortical blindness. These insults may be separated in time so that an apparently unilateral event results in cortical blindness as a result of a corresponding but previously clinically silent contralateral pathology.

Multiple case reports document the varying causes of cortical blindness. The syndrome may be transient after a head injury particularly in children [2]. Transient cortical blindness is also described during preeclampsia [3] and following both cardiac [4] and cerebral angiography [5]. Permanent cortical blindness is usually caused by a vascular event, namely ischaemic stroke (32% of cases in one series) [1]. Although our patient suffered ischaemic damage secondary to critical hypoperfusion, the commonest cause of stroke in this circumstance is thought to be emboli to the posterior circulation [6]. This may be from a central source or a spreading basilar thrombus.

The most important differential diagnosis in cases of cortical blindness is of posterior reversible encephalopathy syndrome (PRES) also known as reversible posterior leukoencephalopathy syndrome (RPLS) [7]. This syndrome of acute metabolic-oedematous capillary leakage is seen in conjunction with a hypertensive encephalopathy and can cause profound visual loss as well as headache, confusion and seizures. It is also a known side effect of immunosuppressive therapy such as cyclosporin. The symptoms are generally reversible with appropriate acute blood pressure management or removal of the causative agent. In addition MR imaging reveals oedema affecting predominantly white matter rather than the mostly cortical damage seen in cases of true cortical blindness.

Prognosis

One case series of patients with cortical blindness reported better visual outcomes in patients under 40, without diabetes or hypertension and with no associated cognitive, language or memory impairment [1]. Lesion location also affects prognosis; in the same series none of the 14 patients with bi-occipital CT abnormalities had good recovery of vision. A separate review of one small cohort [8] suggested that for rehabilitation purposes patients with cortical blindness tend to fall into two distinct groups; total blindness with associated cognitive and behavioural problems and incomplete blindness which may still be severe but has no other associated symptoms. The former group are likely to require permanent nursing care but the latter can be supported to continue living in a community setting with appropriate rehabilitation, as was the case with our patient.

Key Clinical Learning Points
1. Cortical blindness should be suspected in patients with sudden onset of bilateral visual loss but preserved pupillary reflexes, extra ocular movements and normal fundoscopy
2. Imaging aids diagnosis by confirming bilateral pathology in the visual cortices, usually ischaemic stroke
3. PRES is an important diagnosis to exclude
4. Prognosis is poor in terms of the recovery of sight, but patients can recover to independent living with appropriate rehabilitation if they have no associated cognitive deficits or behavioural problems

Key Radiological Learning Points
1. Cortical blindness is associated with bilateral damage to optic tracts or occipital cortex
2. Bilateral borderzone infarctions are associated with cortical blindess
3. PRES causes reversible borderzone ischaemia, and can mimic borderzone infarction

References

1. Aldrich MS, Alessi AG, Beck RW, et al. Cortical blindness: etiology, diagnosis and prognosis. Ann Neurol. 1987;21:149–58.
2. Eldridge PR, Punt J. Transient traumatic cortical blindness in children. Lancet. 1988;331:815–6.
3. Roos NM, Wiegman MJ, Jansonius NM, et al. Visual disturbances in pre-eclampsia. Obstet Gynecol Surv. 2012;67(4):242–50.
4. Alp BN, Bozbuga N, Tuncer MA, et al. Transient cortical blindness after coronary angiography. J Int Med Res. 2009;37(4):1246–51.
5. Clarke TR, Johnson P, Webster D, et al. Transient cortical blindness post angiography- a case report. West Indian Med J. 2011;60(3):357–9.
6. Fisher CM. The posterior cerebral artery syndrome. Can J Neurol Sci. 1986;13:232–9.
7. Hinchey J, Chaves C, Appignani B, et al. A reversible posterior leukoencephalopathy syndrome. N Engl J Med. 1996;334:494–500.
8. Tarek A, Gaber K. Rehabilitation of cortical blindness secondary to stroke. NeuroRehabilitation. 2010;27:321–5.

Chapter 37
Cerebrovascular Disease in Childhood

Georgios Niotakis and Vijeya Ganesan

Clinical History

An 11-year-old caucasian girl was assessed for recurrent episodes of transient hemiparesis affecting right and left sides on separate occasions that had begun whilst she was on holiday in the Canary Islands. Each lasted up to 30 min and she was having 2–3 attacks each week, with complete resolution of symptoms in between. Previous health and development were normal.

Examination

Clinical examination was unremarkable; in particular, cutaneous and cardiovascular examination (including blood pressure) were normal.

Investigations

Brain MRI was initially thought unremarkable but, on review, numerous flow voids were observed in the basal ganglia (Fig. 37.1); MRA of the circle of Willis confirmed occlusive disease of both terminal ICAs. These findings were suggestive of moyamoya disease. Catheter cerebral angiography, undertaken to characterise the

G. Niotakis (✉)
Paediatric Neurology, Great Ormond Street Hospital for Children, London, UK
e-mail: georgios.niotakis@gosh.nhs.uk

V. Ganesan, MRCPCH, MD
Neurosciences Unit, UCL Institute of Child Health, London, UK
e-mail: v.ganesan@ucl.ac.uk

© Springer-Verlag London 2015
S.K. Gill et al. (eds.), *Stroke Medicine: Case Studies from Queen Square*,
DOI 10.1007/978-1-4471-6705-1_37

Fig. 37.1 Axial T1-weighted MRI scan showing multiple flow voids bilaterally in the basal ganglia (*arrow*)

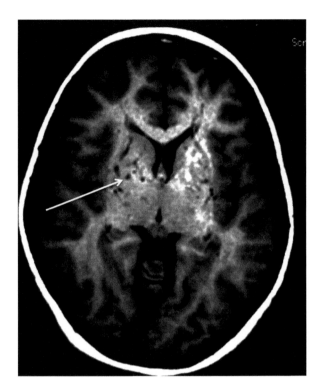

cerebrovascular disease and evaluate the collateral circulation, confirmed this diagnosis, and in addition showed occlusive disease of the left posterior cerebral artery; in the absence of an associated condition, a diagnosis of moyamoya disease was made.

She was treated with low-dose aspirin but continued to have attacks. As the angiogram showed minimal external to internal carotid artery collaterals (Fig. 37.2a), she underwent bilateral surgical revascularisation with pial synangiosis (superficial temporal artery laid onto brain surface). Post-operative angiography showed intracranial supply from the external carotid artery (Fig. 37.2b). Aspirin was discontinued at 18 years of age.

Discussion

Moyamoya disease is an occlusive intracranial arteriopathy of unknown aetiology that involves the terminal internal carotid arteries (ICA) and the proximal MCA and ACA. The posterior circulation (especially posterior cerebral artery) may also be affected. The other characteristic of this pattern of arteriopathy is development of an abnormal network of collateral vessels in the basal ganglia that manifests on catheter angiography as the pathognomonic "puff of smoke" [1].

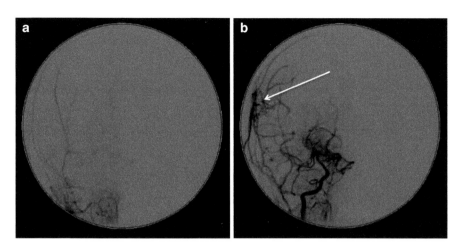

Fig. 37.2 Catheter cerebral angiogram (**a**) pre- and (**b**) post-operatively in patient described above. The external carotid injection in (**a**) does not demonstrate intracranial filling. In (**b**), undertaken after right pial synangiosis, common carotid injection demonstrates both occlusion of the right ICA and intracranial filling via the donor right ECA (*arrow*)

"Moyamoya disease" is by definition idiopathic and bilateral; the term "moyamoya syndrome" is used for cases with an associated diagnosis known to be associated with intracranial arteriopathy [1, 2]. These include:

• genetic conditions (sickle cell disease, neurofibromatosis type 1, Trisomy 21, Alagille syndrome),
• vascular disorders (congenital heart disease, renal artery stenosis, giant cervico-facial haemangiomas, PHACE syndrome),
• other recognised causes (CNS infection, head trauma, previous cranial radiotherapy, SLE, dissection)

Moyamoya disease is endemic in East Asia, with a prevalence of 3.16/100,000 in Japan [1]; linkage studies in these populations have identified several genetic loci [3]. The natural history of moyamoya disease in East Asia is for a high rate of recurrent TIA/ischaemic stroke in childhood. Moyamoya can also present in adult life with TIA or ischaemic stroke. Presentations with cerebral haemorrhage are more common in adulthood than in childhood. It is unclear whether a similarly progressive and aggressive course occurs in people of other ethnicities or in secondary disease born in Asia. Moyamoya disease is less common in Western populations and appears to run a more benign course in many patients, especially in those presenting in adult life. Other presentations include severe focal migraine, seizures, acute chorea and progressive cognitive decline.

The diagnosis of moyamoya disease should be considered in young people with recurrent symptoms of cerebral ischaemia (TIA or stroke) especially if precipitated by hyperventilation (or in hot weather, as in the case above) or if there is an associated condition. Adults with perfusion failure secondary to intracranial occlusive disease often present with "haemodynamic TIAs". These are high frequency attacks often occurring when perfusion falls a critical level, often after taking antihypertensives, or after eating or on exercise. Very often these start with jerking of a limb, mimicking partial epilepsy. Patients with moyamoya disease should be evaluated for the presence of an associated diagnosis. Vascular disease in other systems, especially in the renal arteries, is common [4].

The diagnosis of moyamoya disease is based on radiological criteria (see below), either MRI/MRA or cerebral angiography. Cerebral perfusion studies (MR, Xe-CT, PET, SPECT) can be used to characterise regional cerebral perfusion or cerebrovascular reactivity; however, interpretation of these studies in relation to indications for surgery are not established.

Antiplatelet treatment (aspirin) is usually offered for patients with ischaemic presentations; anticoagulation is generally avoided due to the risk of intracranial haemorrhage from friable collaterals. As the primary mechanism for the ischaemic events is the haemodynamic insufficiency, revascularisation surgery may be considered to provide an alternative collateral circulation. There is a large body of observational evidence to suggest that revascularisation is effective in reducing stroke and TIA [5] but the specific clinical and radiological indications for surgery in individual patients remain controversial. Patients should therefore be referred to a specialised service for moyamoya disease. The AHA childhood stroke guidelines suggest that children with ongoing ischaemic symptoms and evidence of compromised cerebral blood flow or cerebral perfusion reserve should be considered as surgical candidates [2]. Adequate intravenous hydration, maintenance of blood pressure at normal or slightly elevated levels, good pain management (to avert crying) and maintenance of oxygenation are recommended in the perioperative period [2]. If ischaemic symptoms manifest in childhood they commonly improve or resolve during adolescence and into adulthood. Revascularisation is not necessarily indicated in adult patients. Longer-term important management considerations include minimising vascular risk factors (e.g., avoid smoking, manage cholesterol and blood pressure). Blood pressure management is especially important around pregnancy and this may require input from a specialist centre. Revascularisation surgery is not indicated to prevent haemorrhage. The complex nature and location of disease makes endovascular treatments inappropriate.

Key Clinical Learning Points
1. Moyamoya disease should be considered in young patients with recurrent or bilateral stroke or TIA, especially if they have one of the associated conditions
2. Ischaemic symptoms predominate in childhood; haemorrhagic presentations are more common in adults
3. The natural history of the disease is for a high rate of recurrent stroke or TIA
4. Surgical revascularisation is safe and appears effective in preventing recurrent stroke in childhood, although indications are not clearly established
5. Patients commonly have vascular disease in other organs, especially renal arteries

Key Radiological Learning Points
1. Moyamoya is a radiological, rather than clinical, diagnosis
2. Diagnostic criteria on catheter angiography (see Fig. 37.3) are:

   (a) Occlusive disease affecting terminal ICA and/or proximal ACA and/or MCA
   (b) Abnormal vascular networks in the vicinity of the occlusive or stenotic lesions in the arterial phase
   (c) Bilateral involvement in "Moyamoya disease"

3. In addition to the occlusive disease, the presence of more than two flow voids in at least one side of the basal ganglia are sufficient to make the diagnosis on MRI (see Figs. 37.1 and 37.4)
4. Additional radiological features include:

   (a) Multiple infarcts of different age in different arterial territories (see Fig. 37.4)
   (b) diffuse leptomeningeal enhancement on post-contrast MR images or on FLAIR images ("ivy" sign)

5. Catheter angiography is useful to characterise disease morphology, to assess the pattern of collateralisation pre-operatively and to evaluate results of revascularisation surgery (see Fig. 37.2)

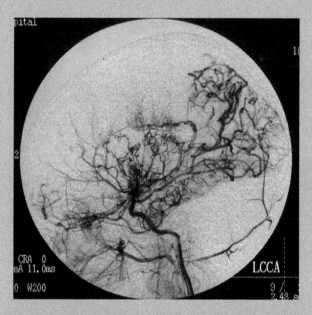

Fig. 37.3 Catheter cerebral angiogram, left CCA injection, lateral view. There is occlusion of the terminal ICA and profuse basal collaterals, as well as collateral supply via the ophthalmic artery. The posterior communicating artery is patent and the CCA injection fills the posterior cerebral artery territory by this route

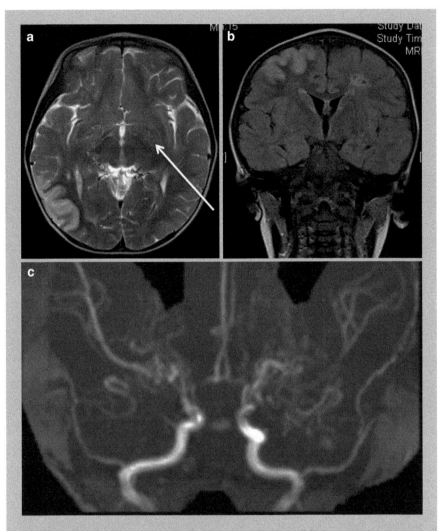

Fig. 37.4 (**a**) Axial T2-weighted (**b**) FLAIR and (**c**) 2D time of flight magnetic resonance angiography of the circle of Willis (*frontal view*) from a 3-year-old child with an acute left hemiparesis. There is an acute right MCA territory infarct with high signal and swelling on T2 and FLAIR; in addition there are cavitated gliotic scars in the white matter of the left hemisphere, representing areas of previous ischaemic injury. The mesh of basal collaterals is apparent in (**a**; see *arrow*). The MRA shows evidence of an arteriopathy affecting terminal ICA and proximal MCA and ACA bilaterally, with profuse proximal "moyamoya" collaterals

References

1. Fukui M. Guidelines for the diagnosis and treatment of spontaneous occlusion of the circle of Willis ("moyamoya" disease). Clin Neurol Neurosurg. 1997;99 Suppl 2:S238–40.
2. Smith ER, Scott RM. Spontaneous occlusion of the circle of Willis in children: pediatric moyamoya summary with proposed evidence-based practice guidelines. A review. J Neurosurg Pediatr. 2012;9:353–60.
3. Achrol AS, Guzman R, Lee M, et al. Pathophysiology and genetic factors in moyamoya disease. Neurosurg Focus. 2009;26(4):E4.
4. Wilsher A, Roebuck D, Ng J, et al. How commonly do children with complex cerebral arteriopathy have renovascular disease? Dev Med Child Neurol. 2013;55(4):335–40.
5. Ng J, Thompson D, Lumley JP, et al. Surgical revascularisation for childhood moyamoya. Childs Nerv Syst. 2012;28:1041–8.

Chapter 38
Recurrent Neurological Symptoms Mistaken as Multiple Sclerosis

Áine Merwick, David J. Werring, and Robert Simister

Clinical History

A 47-year-old lady was seen in neurology outpatients, with a 22-year history of recurrent focal neurological deficits. Her first symptoms occurred at the age of 25 when she experienced high temperatures, a featureless headache, and difficulty walking upstairs and getting up from sitting, along with muscle pains in the proximal legs. Her symptoms lasted for 9 months and then improved.

At age 29, she awoke with double vision, initially in all positions of gaze, but as it improved, the image separation was greater looking towards the left and disappeared on looking to the right; it fully improved within a week. At age 33, she suddenly developed paraesthesia on the sole and on the outer aspect of her right foot. Two weeks later she developed similar symptoms in the left foot, which persisted. Between the age of 33 and 45 she had approximately six discrete episodes of sudden onset of double vision, with horizontal image separation worse looking towards the left and subsequent full resolution. At age 42, whilst at work she suddenly felt unwell and tired, leading her to go to bed. On awakening the next morning, she noticed left sided weakness, without sensory involvement, that took 6 weeks to improve. Five years later, aged 47, she awoke with a sensation that the right side of

Á. Merwick, MB, BMed Sc, MSc, PhD, MRCPI (✉)
Department of Neurology, National Hospital for Neurology and Neurosurgery,
Queen Square, London, UK
e-mail: aine.merwick@uclh.nhs.uk

D.J. Werring, BSc, MBBS, PhD, FRCP
Stroke Research Group, Department of Brain Repair and Rehabilitation, UCL Institute
of Neurology and National Hospital for Neurology and Neurosurgery, London, UK
e-mail: d.werring@ucl.ac.uk

R. Simister, MA, FRCP, PhD
Comprehensive Stroke Service, National Hospital for Neurology and Neurosurgery,
UCLH Trust, London, UK

© Springer-Verlag London 2015   243
S.K. Gill et al. (eds.), *Stroke Medicine: Case Studies from Queen Square*,
DOI 10.1007/978-1-4471-6705-1_38

her body was numb. This gradually improved over 2–3 months, but persisted in her right lower limb. She attended her local hospital and was given a diagnosis of suspected multiple sclerosis. Age 47 she had a further discrete episode of double vision lasting 10 days. She was then referred for a further opinion regarding her recurrent focal neurological symptoms.

In addition to her recurrent focal deficits, she reported headaches which, when present, lasted for several months at a time. There was no variation, exacerbations, movement sensitivity, photophobia, phonophobia, or cranial autonomic features to her headaches. Approximately every 3 months, she also had transient visual symptoms which consist of flashing colours on one side of her vision in both eyes lasting 20–30 min at a time.

. She had no history of rash, iritis, genital or oral ulcerations, or miscarriage. There was a family history of migraine with aura. Her mother reportedly had episodic diplopia but no history of confirmed stroke by age 80. Her brother had been investigated for cardiomyopathy. She smoked cigarettes, but did not report any other vascular risk factors.

Examination

On examination blood pressure at clinic was 168/100, with normal heart sounds. There were no skin lesions. She walked with a spastic gait. Fundi were normal. Eye movements were full with no double vision. She had a supinator catch in the left arm, and increased tone in both lower limbs, worse on the left than on the right with four beats of clonus on the left and three beats of clonus on the right. Power was normal in the right upper limb, but in the left upper limb power was reduced in elbow extension, graded as 4/5 on the MRC scale. She was weak in both legs with hip flexion and foot dorsiflexion on the left both graded 4/5, and foot dorsiflexion graded 4+/5 on the right. Reflexes were brisker on the left side with a crossed adductor response in the left lower limb. The plantar response was extensor on the left and flexor on the right. There were no sensory deficits or cerebellar signs.

Investigations

MRI brain showed subcortical white matter hyperintensities in both hemispheres with normal intracranial vessels. There were regions of abnormal high T2 signal within the mid brain, pons, left thalamus, right corona radiata, right head of caudate and posterior to the left lentiform nucleus. There was a low intensity rim in keeping with some haemosiderin staining at the periphery of some of the lesions. It was concluded that the imaging appearances were consistent with cerebral small vessel disease (Fig. 38.1).

Carotid duplex ultrasound and cardiac monitoring were normal. CSF analysis was also normal, with no oligoclonal bands detected. Echocardiography showed

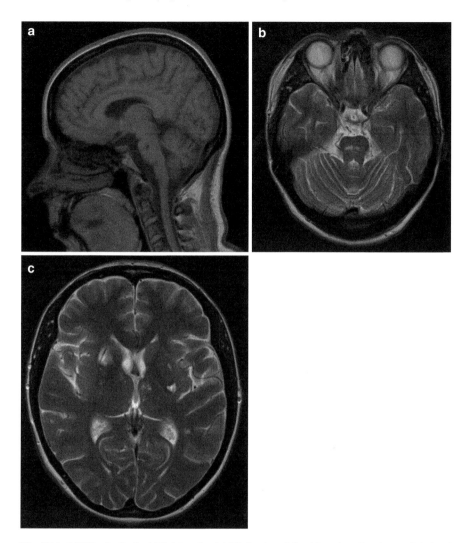

Fig. 38.1 MRI brain Sagittal T1 (**a**) and axial T2 (**b, c**) weighted imaging showing well defined lesions in the pons, left thalamus, right internal capsule/lentiform nucleus and left lentiform nucleus

normal left and right ventricular dimensions and systolic function, with very mild left atrial dilation. Serological tests for thrombophilia, inflammatory markers and autoimmune profiles were negative. Her glomerular filtration rate was 73 mL/min/1.73 sqm. Nerve conduction studies were normal.

The alpha-galactosidase serum enzyme level was 4.7 umol/l/hour (overall reference range 4–21.9 umol/l/hour, Fabry heterozygotes range 0.32–7.4 umol/l/hour). On sequencing the alpha-GAL gene (locus Xq22.1), she was found to be heterozygous for a deletion/insertion mutation between nucleotide 496/497 in exon 3 of the GLA gene, leading to a diagnosis of Fabry's disease.

Discussion

Fabry's disease is an X-linked multi-organ lysosomal storage disease [1]. Deficiency of alpha-galactosidase A activity leads to lysosomal accumulation of glycosphingolipids, predominantly the cerebroside trihexosides in all tissues, including endothelial cells [2]. Patients classically present in childhood with acroparaesthesias, angiokeratomas, hypohydrosis, gastrointestinal symptoms and corneal abnormalities. Without treatment, adult patients may develop multiorgan involvement with cardiomyopathy, neuropathy, renal failure and stroke [3]. Fabry's disease can manifest a variable phenotype, including isolated cerebrovascular disease as well as symptomatic heterozygous females, possibly due to skewed X chromosome lyonisation (X-inactivation) [4–6]. Incidence of alpha-galactosidase A deficiency has been reported as one in 3,000, making it one of the commoner inherited metabolic disorders [7]. Stroke or TIA occur in approximately 13% of affected individuals overall (15% males, 11.5% females) [8]. In a series of 46 patients with Fabry's disease, 44% of adult patients without clinical history of stroke or prior dialysis had evidence of small vessel disease (including white matter hyperintensities on T2-weighted images) on MRI [9]. In one of the first large series, Fabry's disease was reported in up to 5% of cryptogenic stroke patients, but subsequent studies suggest a lower frequency in this group [3, 10].

Increased pulvinar signal intensity on T1-weighted imaging has been reported as a specific feature of Fabry's disease, seen in between 22 and 13.8% of patients. The diagnosis of Fabry's disease in female heterozygotes is especially challenging, as it may mimic sporadic small vessel disease, atherosclerotic cerebrovascular thromboembolic disease, multiple sclerosis (as in this case) or other neuro-inflammatory diseases. Moreover, alpha-galactosidase levels may be normal [5]. Alpha-GAL genetic analysis should be considered in women with atypical presentations of cryptogenic cerebrovascular disease, particularly if there is a previous or family history of unexplained cardiomyopathy, renal failure or neuropathy.

Vascular involvement in Fabry's Disease include disturbances in intraluminal arterial pressure and angioarchitecture leading to dilatation, angiectasia, and dolichoectasia. The vertebrobasilar arteries appear particularly susceptible to dilatational arteriopathy. Small penetrating arteries of the brain frequently become narrowed and occluded [11]. Cerebral infarcts may result from direct vascular occlusion or from distension of branches of the dolichoectatic parent vessels. The precise mechanism of the cerebrovascular involvement is not established. Findings that could contribute to this increased risk include abnormal endothelial dilation via nitric oxide and non-nitric oxide dependent pathways and abnormal endothelial nitric oxide synthase (eNOS) activity [11].

Enzyme replacement therapy is the accepted treatment for symptomatic males and females [6]. Standard vascular secondary prevention measures, including antiplatelet agents, statins and control of hypertension is also recommended in patients with a history of ischaemic stroke.

Key Clinical Learning Points
- Fabry's disease is a cause of ischaemic stroke, particularly in the posterior circulation, and should be considered in younger patients (e.g. <60 years) with MRI evidence of small vessel disease and with no other cause identified for the stroke
- Although Fabry's disease is inherited in an X linked pattern, and stroke typically occurs in male patients, clinically affected females (either homozygous or heterozygous) may also present with stroke
- Serum alphagalactosidase levels may be in the low normal range in heterozygote females
- Stroke can occur without prior systemic manifestations
- Alpha-GAL genetic analysis should be considered in women with atypical presentations of cerebrovascular disease (including those with MRI changes suggesting small vessel disease) or a suggestive family history
- Enzyme replacement therapy may be useful in patients with Fabry's disease

Key Radiological Learning Points
- White matter hyperintensities on T2-weighted MRI in Fabry's disease are non–specific, and the appearances overlap with those of sporadic small vessel disease and can mimic inflammatory conditions
- Hyperintensity of the pulvinar on T1-weighted MRI has been reported as characteristic of Fabry's disease, but has limited sensitivity
- Ischaemic stroke is most frequent in the posterior circulation and in the territories of the penetrating brain stem arteries
- Large arteries are often dilated and tortuous (dolichoectasia), particularly in the posterior circulation

References

1. Eng CM, Desnick RJ. Molecular basis of Fabry disease: mutations and polymorphisms in the human alpha-galactosidase A gene. Hum Mutat. 1994;3:103.
2. Mehta A, Ricci R, Widmer U, et al. Fabry disease defined: baseline clinical manifestations of 366 patients in the Fabry Outcome Survey. Eur J Clin Invest. 2004;34:236–342.
3. Rolfs A, Böttcher T, Zschiesche M, et al. Prevalence of Fabry disease in patients with cryptogenic stroke: a prospective study. Lancet. 2005;366(9499):1794–6.
4. Gregoire SM, Brown MM, Collas DM, et al. Posterior circulation strokes without systemic involvement as the presenting feature of Fabry disease. J Neurol Neurosurg Psychiatry. 2009;80:1414–6.

5. Maier EM, Osterrieder S, Whybra C, et al. Disease manifestations and X inactivation in heterozygous females with Fabry disease. Acta Paediatr. 2006;95(Suppl):30–8.
6. Baehner F, Kapmann C, Whybra C, et al. Enzyme replacement therapy in heterozygous females with Fabry disease: results of a phase IIB study. J Inherit Metab Dis. 2003;26:617–27.
7. Spada M, Pagliardini S, Yasuda M, et al. High incidence of later-onset Fabry disease revealed by newborn screening. Am J Hum Genet. 2006;79:31–40.
8. Ginsberg L, Manara R, Valentine AR, et al. Magnetic resonance imaging changes in Fabry disease. Acta Paediatr Suppl. 2006;95(451):57–62.
9. Reisin RC, Romero C, Marchesoni C, et al. Brain MRI findings in patients with Fabry disease. J Neurol Sci. 2011;305(1–2):41–4.
10. Baptista MV, Ferreira S, Pinho-E-Melo T, et al. Mutations of the GLA gene in young patients with stroke: the PORTYSTROKE study-screening genetic conditions in Portuguese young stroke patients. Stroke. 2010;41(3):431–6.
11. Hilz MJ, Kolodny EH, Brys M, et al. Reduced cerebral blood flow velocity and impaired cerebral autoregulation in patients with Fabry disease. J Neurol. 2004;251(5):564–70.

Chapter 39
Intracerebral Haemorrhage and Oral Anticoagulants

Sumanjit K. Gill and David J. Werring

Clinical History

A 74-year-old man was brought to accident and emergency after collapsing at home. He was seen by his wife to fall to the floor whilst walking across the room. She described an otherwise normal day leading up to this collapse. When she went over to him he was drowsy and was holding his head. She was unable to understand what he was saying. He had a past medical history of hypertension and atrial fibrillation for which he was anticoagulated with warfarin.

Examination

On arrival in hospital, he was drowsy but opened his eyes to voice. His pupils were equal and reactive. He had flaccid weakness of his left arm and leg and was not seen to move this side. The left plantar response was extensor. His blood pressure was elevated at 220/100. The remainder of systemic examination was normal.

S.K. Gill, BSc Hons, MBBS, MRCP (✉)
Education Unit, National Hospital for Neurology and Neurosurgery,
UCL Institute of Neurology, London, UK
e-mail: sumanjit.gill@nhs.net

D.J. Werring, BSc, MBBS, PhD, FRCP
Stroke Research Group, Department of Brain Repair and Rehabilitation,
UCL Institute of Neurology and National Hospital
for Neurology and Neurosurgery, London, UK
e-mail: d.werring@ucl.ac.uk

© Springer-Verlag London 2015   249
S.K. Gill et al. (eds.), *Stroke Medicine: Case Studies from Queen Square*,
DOI 10.1007/978-1-4471-6705-1_39

Investigations and Clinical Progress

ECG showed atrial fibrillation with a controlled ventricular rate and QRS complexes that met the voltage criteria for left ventricular hypertrophy. CT showed an acute haemorrhage in the fronto-parietal region of the right hemisphere (Fig. 39.1). CTA was normal. A diagnosis was made of ICH secondary to warfarin therapy. A point of care testing kit showed that his INR was 3.4 and he was given prothrombin complex concentrate to reverse the warfarin. Labetolol was given as an infusion to reduce his blood pressure, which stabilised at 150/90 20 minutes after starting the infusion.

His scans were discussed with a neurosurgical centre and he was transferred there for monitoring of intracranial pressure. He then deteriorated and hydrocephalus was found on a repeat CT head. An external ventricular drain was therefore inserted, but could be removed after 4 days. He was transferred to a rehabilitation unit and upon discharge he was able to transfer from bed to chair and communicate his needs. A decision was made not to restart anticoagulation due to the risk of another intracerebral haemorrhage.

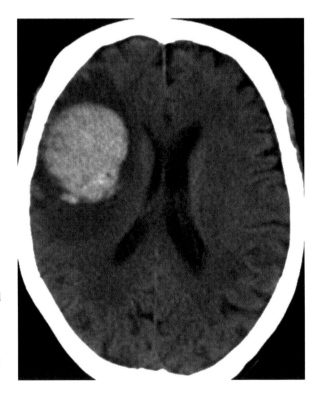

Fig. 39.1 Unenhanced axial CT image showing a large acute haemorrhage in the right hemisphere fronto-temporal region with some deformity of the right lateral ventricle

Discussion

ICH may occur secondary to an identified underlying structural cause, for example an aneurysm or AVM. However, in about 80% of cases, ICH is 'primary' i.e. the cause is not seen on conventional vascular imaging. However, the majority of 'primary' haemorrhages are actually secondary to underlying disease of cerebral small vessels, commonly hypertensive vasculopathy or amyloid angiopathy. Hypertension is potentially an aggravating factor in all types of ICH; recent data suggests that peak levels or variability may be more important than average baseline blood pressure.

Intracerebral haemorrhage has a 30-day mortality of 55% with half these deaths occurring in the first two days [1]. It is therefore important that these patients are closely monitored in the acute phase and clinicians should be responsive to any deterioration. The main cause of acute deterioration is raised intracranial pressure either from the initial bleed, secondary to haematoma expansion or from hydrocephalus, as in this case. Perihaematomal oedema can also exacerbate the situation. In the subacute and rehabilitation phase other factors such as venous thromboembolism, sepsis and hypertension become more prominent complications of ICH.

Haematoma expansion is an independent predictor of poor outcome, and affects 70% of patients in the first 24 hours [2]. Predictors of an increase in haematoma size include a large volume of the initial ICH, heterogeneity of haematoma density (implying a slowly expanding bleed), contrast extravasation ("spot sign") [2, 3] and anticoagulant or antiplatelet use. Intraventricular extension of a haemorrhage is also a strong predictor of poor prognosis.

Perihaematomal oedema develops in the first 24 hours after onset and evolves over the following days to reach a peak in the second week after onset. The oedema occurs as a result of a leakage of protein and electrolytes across the blood brain barrier; thrombin production and activation of the clotting cascade also produces an inflammatory response in the surrounding tissue. There is no evidence for any useful benefit of steroid therapy and measures to manage the raised ICP are initially conservative e.g. head elevation to 30°, hyperventilation to reduce partial pressures of CO_2 and close monitoring. Hydrocephalus may require temporary or permanent drainage.

ICH associated with oral anticoagulation (OAC-ICH) is one of the serious side effects of these drugs with mortality up to 60% making them a particularly lethal form of stroke [4, 5]. The increase in mortality is attributable to continued haematoma expansion, so the initial aim of management is to reverse the coagulopathy as quickly as possible. Typically, prothrombin complex concentrate is used if the OAC is warfarin, although there are no randomized data to confirm its effectiveness. In the case of the newer oral anticoagulants there is no scope for reversal at present, but in severe cases haemofiltration may be considered; recombinant clotting factors have emerging potential as future antidotes. Strong predictors of OAC-ICH are advanced age, hypertension, and previous ischaemic stroke. There is an association with bleeding prone angiopathies including cerebral microbleeds [6]. The annual incidence of OAC-ICH in this group may be up 1.8% per year [5]. Unfortunately, risk factors for microbleeds overlap with the group that is most likely to benefit from anticoagulation, making it difficult to assess the risk-benefit balance when considering initiating anticoagulation. As the causes of OAC-ICH and spontaneous ICH overlap, it is likely they have the same aetiology with anticoagulation acting as an exacerbating factor. A proportion of patients with OAC-ICH would presumably have had a spontaneous ICH independent of anticoagulation, but even then it is likely that the anticoagulation increases the size of the bleed and there is no doubt that the outcome of OAC-ICH is worse than that of spontaneous ICH.

The only intervention that might improve outcome of ICH at the time of writing is rapid blood pressure lowering within 6 hours of onset to a target of 140 mmHg systolic, as suggested by the INTERACT-2 trial [7]. However, there are on-going trials of recombinant Factor VIIa and tranexamic acid among other treatments and this advice may change in the near future.

The STICH II trial [8] has confirmed that there is no overall benefit from early evacuation of clot as opposed to medical management alone of ICH, although possible benefit was suggested where the haemorrhage is lobar and superficial (within 1 cm of the brain surface). Outcomes from trials of clot aspiration techniques using lytic agents are awaited. Nevertheless, most patients will benefit from a neurosurgical opinion as acute obstructive hydrocephalus may require an external ventricular drain in the first instance, as in this case, or to monitor the high risk patient in case life saving intervention is required.

A list of possible causes of intraparenchymal intracerebral haemorrhage is given in Box 39.1.

Box 39.1: Some Causes of Intraparenchymal Intracerebral Haemorrhage
1. Hypertensive arteriopathy
2. Arteriovenous malformation
3. Cerebral Amyloid angiopathy
4. Intracranial neoplasm
5. Haemorrhagic transformation of ischaemic stroke
6. Cerebral Venous sinus thrombosis
7. Vasculitis
8. Aneurysmal rupture
9. Eclampsia
10. Vasculitis
11. Cocaine abuse

Key Clinical Learning Points
1. ICH is a condition with a high mortality especially in the acute phase – an ABCDE approach should be followed and anticoagulation, if present, promptly reversed
2. It might be beneficial to lower raised blood pressure quickly and effectively
3. Worsening in the clinical condition could signal haematoma expansion or perihaematomal oedema and the patient should be rescanned
4. Angiography should be performed to look for any evidence of an underlying structural cause of ICH in discussion with a multidisciplinary vascular team

Key Radiological Learning Points
1. Intraventricular extension of haemorrhage is a sign of a poor prognosis
2. A visible spot sign on CT angiography signals that there is still active bleeding and is a strong predictor of poor outcome

References

1. Balami JS, Buchan AM. Complications of intracerebral haemorrhage. Lancet Neurol. 2012;11(1):101–18.
2. Davis SM, Broderick J, Hennerici M, et al. Hematoma growth is a determinant of mortality and poor outcome after intracerebral hemorrhage. Neurology. 2006;66:1175–81.
3. Delgado Almandoz JE, Yoo AJ, Stone MJ, et al. The spot sign score in primary intracerebral hemorrhage identifies patients at highest risk of in-hospital mortality and poor outcome among survivors. Stroke. 2010;41:54–60.
4. Hart RG, Boop B, Anderson DC. et al. Oral anticoagulants and intracerebral haemorrhage: facts and hypotheses. Stroke. 1995;26:1471–7.
5. Stenier T, Rosand J, Diringer M. et al. Intracerebral haemorrhage associated with oral anticoagulant therapy. Stroke. 2006;37:256–62.
6. Lovelock C, Cordonnier C, Naka H, et al. Antithrombotic drug use, cerebral microbleeds and intracerebral haemorrhage. Stroke. 2010;41:1222–8.
7. Anderson CS, Heeley E, Huang Y, et al. Rapid blood pressure lowering in patients with acute intracerebal haemorrhage. N Engl J Med. 2013;368:2355–65.
8. Mendelow AD, Gregson BA, Rowan EN, et al. Early surgery versus initial conservative treatment in patients with spontaneous supratentorial lobar intracerebral haematomas (STICH II): a randomised trial. Lancet. 2013;382(9890):397–408.

Chapter 40
Choked in the Night

Sumanjit K. Gill and David Collas

Clinical History

A 50-year-old man was woken at night by a choking sensation, in a cold sweat. He felt unwell but went back to sleep. On waking the next morning, he had difficulty drinking his tea and swallowing toast. During a shower, he was conscious that he could not feel the temperature of the hot water on the right side of his body. His daughter, an optician, commented that his left eye looked odd, with a slightly drooping eyelid. He gave a past medical history of uncomplicated Type 1 Diabetes Mellitus.

Examination

On examination, he gave his history with a slightly croaking voice. Examination of his eyes showed a left Horner's syndrome, characterised by mild drooping of the left eyelid and inequality of the pupils, which was only detectable in dim light when the right pupil dilated, but the left did not. There was also a detectable deviation of the soft palate to the right when elevated. The other cranial nerves were intact. Sensation on the right side of the body was slightly reduced to pin prick but there was no reduction in sensation in the face on either side. A test of swallowing provoked a prolonged fit of coughing.

S.K. Gill, BSc Hons, MBBS, MRCP (✉)
Education Unit, National Hospital for Neurology and Neurosurgery,
UCL Institute of Neurology, London, UK
e-mail: sumanjit.gill@nhs.net

D. Collas, BSc, MB, BS FRCP
Stroke Medicine, Watford General Hospital, Watford, UK

© Springer-Verlag London 2015

S.K. Gill et al. (eds.), *Stroke Medicine: Case Studies from Queen Square*,
DOI 10.1007/978-1-4471-6705-1_40

Investigations and Clinical Progress

An initial diagnosis of a brainstem vascular event in the medulla was made, possibly a variant of lateral medullary syndrome, but there was only mild dizziness without true vertigo, and none of the other expected symptoms of the lateral medullary symptoms such as vomiting, hiccups, cerebellar ataxia or nystagmus.

CT brain showed no abnormality. MRI showed an acute infarct in the left medulla. DWI and ADC map images (Fig. 40.1) confirmed that this was an acute infarct and FLAIR sequences (Fig. 40.2) confirmed there were no other lesions.

He was initially managed nil-by-mouth and a naso-gastric tube was inserted for fluid and nutrition. However, his swallowing recovered within 3 days, allowing the feeding tube to be removed.

After 3 months, the patient returned to full-time employment. His speech had fully recovered but he continued to experience very mild subjective sensory loss, scoring 1 on the mRS. His temperature sensation on the right remained impaired to the extent that he reported that if he put both hands round a hot kettle he could not appreciate the heat with his right hand. If he went outside in the cold, only the left side of his body felt cold, while his right side might have a slight sensation of warmth.

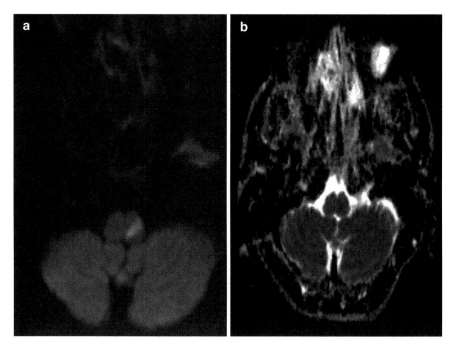

Fig. 40.1 Axial B1000 diffusion weighted sequence (**a**) and ADC map (**b**) confirming a left sided medullary infarct

Fig. 40.2 Axial T2 FLAIR image of left medullary infarct

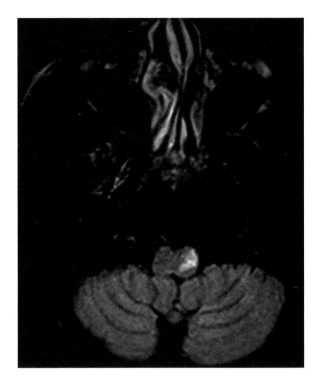

Discussion

The territory affected by this infarct in the left lateral medulla covers the nucleus ambiguous and the spino-thalamic and descending sympathetic tracts, accounting for the dysphagia, dysphonia, ipsilateral weakness of palatal elevation, Horner's syndrome and contralateral pain and temperature loss [1, 2]. This specific variety of lateral medullary syndrome is known as Avelli's syndrome, after the first report in a case series in 1891 by George Avelli, a German laryngologist [3]. A slightly more rostral lesion may involve some facial nerve fascicles and produce an additional facial palsy of a lower motor neurone type.

A larger infarct extending to adjacent territory will produce a wider cluster of symptoms and signs, as detailed in the history of another patient given in Fig. 40.3. The brain stem is supplied by small perforating arteries, which are branches of the vertebral and basilar arteries. Occlusions of these often present with complex crossed deficits and cranial nerve palsies which are classified as various syndromes. An outline of these is given in Table 40.1. These can be difficult to recognise, but the history of a sudden onset should give a pointer towards a vascular cause.

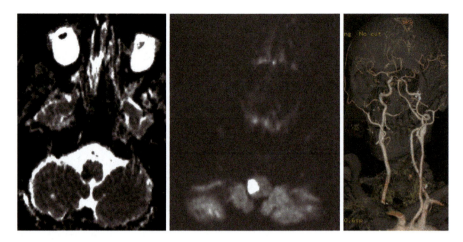

Fig. 40.3 Another brainstem syndrome. ADC map and DWI confirming an acute infarct in the right medulla with CTA displaying an occluded right vertebral artery. A 56-year-old male suddenly became dizzy and unsteady, with loss of sensation over his right side, change in his voice (dysphonia) followed by loss of speech, and hiccup. His vascular risk factors were Type II Diabetes Mellitus, hypertension, and smoking. On examination, he had profound dysarthria and nystagmus on leftward gaze. CT was normal and he received thrombolysis for presumed ischaemic stroke. MRI demonstrated a large infarct in the right lateral medulla, and an absence of the normal flow void in the right vertebral artery, indicating occlusion. CTA confirmed that only a short segment of the right vertebral artery was patent, and given the headache and his job as a roofer, vertebral artery dissection from minor trauma was considered the most likely cause of his stroke on the background of atheroma caused by his diabetes, hypertension and smoking

Table 40.1 Main brainstem syndromes with the corresponding site of lesion and clinical manifestations

Eponymous syndrome	Site of infarct	Arterial supply	Clinical features
Marie Foix syndrome	Lateral pontine	Anterior inferior cerebrallar artery	Ipsilateral ataxia
			Contralateral weakness
			Contralateral hemisensory loss
Wallenberg syndrome	Lateral medullary	Posterior inferior cerebellar artery	Ipsilateral horners syndrome
			Ipsilateral nystagmus
			Ipsilateral ataxia
			Ipsilateral facial sensory loss
			Dysphagia
			Vertigo
			Contralateral hemisensory loss
Foville syndrome	Inferior medial pontine	Basillar	Contralateral weakness
			Ipsilateral weakness of the face
			Ipsilateral 6th CN palsy
Dejerine syndrome	Medial medullary	Basilar or anterior spinal	Contralateral weakness
			Hemisensory loss
			Ipsilateral tongue weakness

Table 40.1 (continued)

Eponymous syndrome	Site of infarct	Arterial supply	Clinical features
Raymond syndrome	Ventral pontine	Paramedian branches of basilar	Ipsilateral 6th CN palsy
			Contralateral weakness
Millard Gubler syndrome	Ventral pontine	Basilar artery	Contralateral weakness
			Contralateral sensory loss
			Ipsilateral tongue weakness

Key Clinical Learning Points

1. Choking spontaneously at night with sweating are unusual symptoms with a wide differential diagnosis: paroxysmal nocturnal dyspnoea, nightmares, laryngospasm, pharyngeal pouch, asthma – which might be difficult to channel into a diagnosis. A full history and examination is required to narrow the possibilities

2. Horner's syndrome is a subtle sign, which is rarely noticed by the patient, as in this case. It must be specifically looked for during examination: this is best done in dim light so that the unaffected pupil dilates, making the asymmetry obvious

3. The close clustering of contiguous structures in the brainstem results in a variety of different syndromes – the important part of diagnosis after hearing a full history is to look carefully for additional physical signs pointing to a brain stem origin (e.g. abnormal elevation of the palate), then seek radiological confirmation

4. The hallmark of brain stem syndromes is crossed signs i.e. signs in the limbs on one side of the body in combination with cranial nerve palsies on the contralateral side; if these are found, then an MRI is the investigation of choice because a small or early posterior fossa infarct can be missed on CT, as in this case

Key Radiological Learning Points

1. Brainstem lesions with significant symptoms and signs may be small and visible in only one slice on MRI scanning – they may be missed unless the clinician directs the radiologist to the site of the suspected lesion

2. Angiography may be useful if the parent lesion is in a vertebral artery, but when the occlusion is in a small perforating artery, the vascular appearances may be normal

3. The appearance and sudden onset should enable a distinction to be made between vascular lesions in the brainstem and other pathology, e.g. inflammatory lesions

References

1. Kataoka S, Hori A, Hirose G, et al. Avelli's syndrome: the neurological-topographical correlation. Eur Neurol. 2001;45:292–3.
2. Takizawa S, Shinohara Y. Magnetic resonance imaging in Avelli's syndrome. J Neurol Neurosurg Psychiatry. 1996;61:17.
3. Imperatori CJ. Syndrome of Avellis: a report of 3 cases. Arch Otolaryngol. 1925;1(3):277–82. doi:10.1001/archotol.1925.00560010293003.

Abbreviations

12L ECG	12-lead electrocardiogram
αβ2GPI	Anti beta 2 glycoprotein I
α-GAL	Alpha galactosidase gene
A&E	Accident and emergency
ABCD2	Clinical risk prediction tool based on Age, Blood pressure, Clinical features, Disability and the presence of Diabetes Mellitus
ACA	Anterior cerebral artery
ACE	Angiotensin-converting enzyme
ACE-R	Addenbrooke's Cognitive Examination
aCL	Anticardiolipin
ACTA 2	Smooth muscle specific isoform alpha actin
ACST-2	Asymptomatic Carotid Surgery Trial −2
ADC	Apparent diffusion coefficient
AHA	American Heart Association
AHI	Apnoea Hypopnea Index
AIS	Arterial ischaemic stroke
AF	Atrial fibrillation
AMTS	Abbreviated mental test score
ANA	Antinuclear antibody
ANCA	Anti-neutrophil cytoplasmic antibody
AP	Antero-posterior orientation
APS	Antiphospholipid syndrome
APTT	Activated partial thromboplastin time
ArmA	Arm Activity Measure
AVM	Arteriovenous malformation
BASICS	Basilar Artery International Cooperation Study
BCSH	British Committee for Standards in Haematology
BMI	Body mass index
BP	Blood pressure

CAA	Cerebral amyloid angiopathy
CADASIL	Cerebral Autosomal-Dominant Arteriopathy with Stroke Like Episodes and Leukencephalopathy
CCA	Common carotid artery
CCP	Anti citrullinated protein antibody
CDC	Centre for Disease Control
CDUS	Carotid Doppler ultrasound
CEA	Carotid endarterectomy
CHA_2DS_2-VASc	Calculates stroke risk in those with atrial fibrillation
CI	Confidence interval
CMV	Cytomegalovirus
CNS	Central nervous system
CO_2	Carbon dioxide
cPAP	Continuous positive airway pressure
CRP	C-reactive protein
CMIA	HIV testing
CNS	Central nervous system
COPD	Chronic obstructive pulmonary disease
CSF	Cerebrospinal fluid
CT	Computerised tomography
CTA	Computed tomography angiography
CTV	Computerised tomography venography
CVT	Cerebral venous thrombosis
DC	Direct current
DHC	Decompressive hemicraniectomy
DNA	Deoxyribonucleic acid
dsDNA	Double-stranded DNA
DRVVT	Dilute Russell's viper venom time
DVT	Deep venous thrombosis
DWI	Diffusion weighted images
ECA	External carotid artery
EC-IC	Extra cranial–intracranial
ECST-2	European carotid artery trial–2
EDS	Excessive daytime sleepiness
EEG	Electro encephalogram
EIA	Enzyme immunoassay
EMG	Electromyography
ENAs	Extractable nuclear antigens
eNOS	Endothelial nitric oxide synthase
ESS	Epworth sleepiness score
ESR	Erythrocyte sedimentation rate
FBC	Full blood count
FCR	Flexor carpi radialis
FCU	Flexor carpi ulnaris
FDS	Flexor digitorum superficialis

FFT	Free floating thrombus
FLAIR	Fluid-attenuated inversion recovery sequences
FTA	Fluorescein treponemal antibody
GABA	Gamma aminobutyric acid
GCS	Glasgow Coma Scale
GP	General practitioner
H&E stain	Haematoxylin eosin stain
HA	Hemianopic alexia
HASU	Hyperacute stroke unit
Hb	Haemoglobin
HbF	Foetal haemoglobin
HbS%	The proportion of sickle cell haemoglobin
HbSS	Sickle cell disease
HBV	Hepatitis B virus
HCV	Hepatitis C virus
HDL	High density lipoprotein
HHT	Hereditary haemorrhagic telengectasia
HIV	Human immunodeficiency virus
HLA	Human leukocyte antigen
HZO	Herpes zoster opthalmicus
IAT	Intra-arterial thrombolysis
ICA	Internal carotid artery
ICH	Intracerebral haemorrhage
ICP	Intracranial pressure
INR	International normalised ratio
IOP	Intra ocular pressure
ITU	Intensive care unit
IUD	Intra uterine device
IV	Intravenous
IVT	Intravenous thrombolysis
JAK2	Janus kinase 2
LA	Lupus anticoagulant
LMWH	Low molecular weight heparin
LVH	Left ventricular hypertrophy
MCA	Middle cerebral artery
MCP	Metacarpophalangeal joint
MELAS syndrome	Mitochondrial encephalomyopathy, lactic acidosis, and stroke-like episodes syndrome
MHA	Microhaemagglutination assay
MI	Myocardial infarction
MMCAS	Malignant middle cerebral artery syndrome
MMSE	Mini mental score examination
MoCA	Montreal Cognitive Examination
MRA	Magnetic resonance angiography
MRC Score	Medical research council score

MRI	Magnetic resonance imaging
mRS	Modified Rankin Scale
MTS	Mental test score
MS	Multiple sclerosis
NIHSS	National Institute of Health Stroke Scale
NOAC	New oral anticoagulant
NSAIDs	Non-steroidal anti-inflammatory drugs
OAC-ICH	Oral anticoagulant-associated intracerebral haemorrhage
OSA	Obstructive sleep apnoea
PCA	Posterior cerebral artery
PDA	Patent ductus arteriosus
PCR	Polymerase chain reaction
PHACE	Posterior Fossa Malformations-Hemangiomas-Arterial Anomalies-Cardiac Defects-Eye Abnormalities-Sternal Cleft and Supraumbilical Raphe Syndrome
PE	Pulmonary embolus
PEG	Percutaneous endoscopic gastrostomy
PET	Positron emission tomography
PFO	Patent foramen ovale
PICA	Posterior inferior cerebellar artery
PIP	Proximal interphalangeal joint
PoCA	Posterior communicating artery
PRES	Posterior reversible encephalopathy syndrome
PRKAR1A	cAMP-dependent protein kinase type I-alpha regulatory subunit
PT	Prothrombin time
RAPS	Rivaroxaban in anti-phospholipid syndrome
RCC	Red cell count
RCT	Randomised control trials
RCVS	Reversible cerebral vasoconstriction syndrome
RoPE	Risk of Paradoxical Embolus Score
RPLS	Reversible posterior leukoencephalopathy syndrome
RPR	Rapid plasma reagin
RR	Respiratory rate
rtPA	Recombinant tissue plasminogen activator
SAH	Subarachnoid haemorrhage
SCD	Sickle cell disease
SDB	Sleep-disordered breathing
SLE	Systemic lupus erythematosis
SMC	Smooth muscle cells
SPECT	Single-photon emission computed tomography
STA-MCA	Superficial temporal artery to middle cerebral artery
SWI	Susceptibility weighted imaging
T2* GRE	T2-weighted gradient echo sequences
TAAD	Thoracic artery aneurysms and dissection

TB	Tuberculosis (mycobacterium)
TCD	Transcranial Doppler
TIA	Transient ischaemic attack
TFT	Thyroid function test
TGA	Transient global amnesia
TOE	Transoesophageal echocardiogram
TPPA	*Treponema pallidum* particle agglutination assay
UCL	University College London
UH	Unfractionated heparin
VA	Vertebral artery
VDRL	Veneral Disease Research Laboratory Test
VKA	Vitamin K antagonists
VTE	Venous thromboembolism
VZV	Varicella zoster virus
WCC	White cell count
Xe CT	Xenon-enhanced CT scan

Index

CPI Antony Rowe

Chippenham, UK

2016-12-21 21:43